FPA Contraceptive handbook

The essential reference guide for family planning and other health professionals

Toni Belfield

Head of Information and Research

Family Planning Association

Published by the Family Planning Association
27-35 Mortimer Street, London WIN 7RJ

British Library Cataloguing in Publication Data
A catalogue record for this book is available from the
British Library

ISBN 0 903289 77 6

Designed by Andrew Haig & Associates
Geoffrey Haddon, Heleen Franken
Design consultant Peter Gill
Illustrations by Sean MacGarry
Cover photograph by Paul Mattock

Printed in Great Britain by
The College Hill Press Limited

Contents

**Acknowledge-
ments**

Thank you to the following who gave their time to provide helpful comments and advice: John Guillebaud (Professor of Family Planning and Reproductive Health Care – Medical Director, Margaret Pyke Centre), Michael Orme (Professor of Clinical Pharmacology, University of Liverpool), and David Back (Reader – Department of Pharmacology and Therapeutics, University of Liverpool).

A special thank you to Jane Urwin (FPA Medical Information Officer), Jane Hobden (FPA Publications Officer), Lucy Owens (FPA Publicity/Editorial Assistant) and Nina Behrman (freelance editor).

Foreword

I am delighted to be able to introduce to you the *FPA Contraceptive handbook*. A clear, comprehensive guide to contraceptive methods and services, it will be an invaluable reference book for family planning and other health professionals. Detailed information is presented in an accessible manner, making it a convenient resource for those working in all kinds of settings.

Contraception is an area which is constantly changing and this book covers the newest as well as current methods. With over 60 years' experience in family planning, the FPA is ideally placed to produce a resource which answers the needs of the many thousands of professionals and consumers with whom it speaks every year. This book makes a welcome addition to those existing in the field.

David Bromham
Chair of the Faculty of Family Planning and Reproductive Health Care of the Royal College of Obstetricians and Gynaecologists

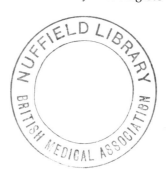

Introduction

This handbook is intended for family planning professionals and other health professionals who work within the area of reproductive and sexual health. *All* professionals work within their own professional codes of conduct and these codes govern daily practice.

The handbook aims to provide a convenient and comprehensive reference guide to family planning methods and services. In addition it addresses other areas of reproductive and sexual health such as pre-pregnancy care, sexually transmitted infections and abortion.

Knowing about contraception and being able to make informed choices about methods is a fundamental issue and contributes greatly to the health and well being of us all. But, *how* contraception is *considered, discussed* and, more importantly, *delivered* will determine just how well it is accepted *and* used. Recognising that these all interrelate and acknowledging the need to improve the uptake and use of contraceptive methods is as important as recognising that choice of contraception is inextricably linked with emotional and sexual well-being. It is impossible to talk about family planning and contraception without addressing sexuality – the two are inseparable. Professionals working in these areas need to recognise and acknowledge that because of this, contraception continues to be a source of considerable embarrassment and anxiety for both women and men, and this has implications for its uptake and usage. Importantly, this embarrassment, can have an inhibiting effect on people's willingness to seek information and advice from professionals.

Contraception, sexual and reproductive health, more that any other branch of medicine, is an area where a partnership between the public and professionals is vital. The provision of full, accurate and objective information contributes to that partnership and through such information truly informed choices and decisions can be made.

A final note

This handbook cannot and is not intended to replace appropriate training. Family planning and sexual health are not wholly medical issues. The FPA's experience of more than 60 years working with family planning providers, and of handling more than 200,000 enquiries yearly from professionals and the public, confirms the need for all those working in the field of family planning and sexual health to have appropriate clinical *and* non-clinical training. This should involve an awareness of sexuality, an exploration of values and attitudes and the development of communication and active listening skills. Such training will enable professionals to work with women and men of all ages, abilities, cultures, faith or values and to respond appropriately.

The FPA can provide full information on all aspects of family planning, contraceptive methods, sexual and reproductive health; including service provision within the UK. The FPA also produces a full range of leaflets and publications for the general public and professionals on the different contraceptive methods. See 'Recommended reading' on page 160.

Family planning services

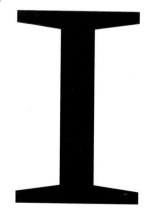

The need for family planning and reproductive health services

Family planning and reproductive health are essential parts of preventive health care, and sexual health is an important area of public health. Family planning was defined as an essential component of primary health care in the Alma-Ata Declaration of 1978. In addition family planning has been identified as a key area in English Department of Health's document, *The health of the nation* where it states:

'Planned parenthood provides benefits for the health of individuals, families and communities. Family planning services aim to promote this by providing access to contraception, sterilisation and advice on unplanned pregnancy. Additionally, education, counselling and health promotion can enable prospective parents to choose healthy lifestyles and increase the chances that their children will be wanted and healthy. Delaying and spacing pregnancies and limiting family size contributes to the physical and mental health of mothers and children and general family well-being.

Purchasers should be aware of the potential of family planning services to improve health by the prevention of unplanned pregnancies and by other health promotion strategies and should work with all appropriate agencies to ensure that services available to local people are complementary and meet identified needs.'

Family planning embraces far more than just the methods of contraception; it is part of and includes reproductive health. Family planning aims to enable people to choose whether and when to have children. This includes birth control, planning a baby, timing conception, spacing births and infertility advice and help. Family planning encompasses emotional well-being and affects the individual's enjoyment of his or her own sexuality.

The FPA believes that sexual health, sexuality and family planning are issues of national concern. They directly affect the health and well-being of present and future generations and must have a place both in public health strategies and in health promotion work. Access to information and education on sexual health and family planning is essential. Those providing family planning services should recognise that an individual's requirements will vary depending on gender, age, class, race, culture or disability, and that services should be flexible enough to meet those different needs.

Comprehensive and free NHS family planning services

Until the mid-1970s the FPA developed and ran well over 1,000 UK family planning clinics. Following the National Health Service Reorganisation Act 1973 (which came into force in 1974) all contraceptive services became free to women and men within the National Health Service. As a result the FPA's family planning clinics were incorporated into the NHS. Family planning clinics are now run by the district health authorities in England and Wales and by the health boards in Scotland and Northern Ireland. In 1975, general practitioners also agreed to provide free family planning services and most GPs now offer contraceptive advice and methods, though not necessarily all methods (for example, condoms).

Women and men are free to choose where they go for family planning advice and supplies. This applies to anyone irrespective of age, sex or marital status. Free contraceptive services are available from GPs, family planning clinics, in hospitals, through a domiciliary service, some genitourinary medicine clinics or from voluntary agencies such as Brook Advisory Centres.

At present, over 25 per cent of women and men receive family planning advice and supplies from health authority community clinics, and over 70 per cent from GP services. Although many people are happy to obtain family planning advice and supplies from their GP, community-based clinic and domiciliary services provided by the local health authority are vital for a number of reasons. Most important of these are choice and the recognition that health authority services complement, rather than duplicate those services provided by GPs. Commitment to choice and complementary provision underpin government policy, as stated in the following extract taken from Executive Letter (EL(90)MB115). This letter was sent by the Department of Health to all regional general managers in June 1990, drawing attention to previous family planning guidelines and expressing concern about reductions in health authority family planning clinic services.

'Government policy remains that people should be free to choose their source of contraceptive advice and that health authority family planning services complement, rather than duplicate, those which GPs provide. Choice is important to ensure that all those who wish to use this service can do so.'

Further communications and guidelines were issued in 1991 and 1992 to ensure that purchasers of family planning services (DHAs and FHSAs) address aspects of the quality and range of family planning services in the UK. With all the changes in the NHS at present, it is not possible to predict how the provision of family planning services will change in the future.

Many people are apprehensive about seeking advice and information on this subject. Health professionals can therefore play an important role by providing relevant information and enabling women and men to use family planning services more effectively. Delivery of services whether through general practice or through community clinics are an important area of contraceptive compliance. Accessible services are important and professionals have a responsibility to look closely at the services they offer to the public in order to ensure that family planning and sexual health services are:

▶ appropriately targeted
▶ effective
▶ efficient
▶ of good quality

The FPA can provide detailed information on all contraceptive methods, family planning clinic services and reproductive help services in the UK (see 'The role of the UK FPA' on page 16). Family planning and health professionals may contact the FPA direct or refer enquirers to the FPA for information. Information about family planning services can also be obtained from:

▶ the District Health Authority (clinics only)
▶ the Family Health Services Authority (family doctors only)
▶ local health centre/hospital
▶ midwife, health visitor
▶ post office/public library
▶ telephone directory
▶ local information centres or health lines.

Family planning services

Recognising that family planning embraces more than just the mechanics of contraception and includes reproductive and sexual health means that this should be reflected in all family planning services that are offered. The following guidelines should be considered:

Family planning provision should include:

▶ a full range of contraceptive methods, including condoms and postcoital contraception
▶ counselling and referral for male and female sterilisation
▶ pregnancy testing and counselling for unplanned pregnancy
▶ pre-pregnancy advice
▶ advice and help with regard to sexual health and 'safer sex'
▶ help or referral for sexual and relationship problems
▶ well woman/well man services
▶ advice, treatment or referral for sexually transmitted diseases (STDs)
▶ advice, help or referral for infertility
▶ advice, help or referral for the menopause and premenstrual tension (PMT)

Service provision should include:

▶ accessible and flexible clinic services
▶ sufficient time for family planning consultations, *especially* the first visit
▶ an assurance of *confidentiality* in visits, communications and record keeping
▶ a choice (where possible) of male or female doctor
▶ appropriate referral mechanisms

Training

▶ ensure *all* staff (including reception and clerical staff) are appropriately trained

Information

▶ always provide standardised, complete, up-to-date and objective information, ie the information *you* yourself would expect to receive
▶ use suitable up-to-date language that both enables and informs, eg *do* talk about IUDs, progestogen-only pills, natural family planning and postcoital (or emergency) contraception, do *not* talk about coils, mini-pills, rhythm methods or morning-after contraception
▶ always discuss risks *and* benefits
▶ recognise people are not always comfortable and may not feel able to ask questions. 'Check out' information needs of clients
▶ *always* provide written information that backs up and reinforces any verbal advice
▶ provide information about services so people know about them

NHS family planning clinics

Family planning clinics provide a choice of birth control methods and advice, and in addition provide help on many related matters.

Procedures at clinics

At the first visit to a family planning clinic the client's name, address and age are noted and the name and address of their general practitioner. Permission should always be sought at this stage as to whether or not a GP may be contacted, and how a client can be contacted by the clinic. The doctor or nurse at the clinic should discuss the various methods of contraception with the client and help choose a suitable one. Relevant details of the client's medical history and family medical history are noted. Blood pressure and weight may be checked and an internal examination may be carried out, but this can sometimes be postponed to a second or later visit. The client should then be taught how to use the chosen method, given a leaflet to take home as a reminder, and also a follow-up appointment. Contraceptive supplies are provided at the clinic.

If oral contraception, the intrauterine device (IUD), post-coital contraception or sterilisation is chosen, the client's own doctor will usually be informed, but *not without* the person's permission. Cervical cytology results are also sent to a client's GP.

General practitioner family planning provision

The majority of general practitioners provide a contraceptive service. A person may attend their own GP or choose to go to another GP who offers a family planning service *without* a referral.

Doctors can arrange for clients to go elsewhere (eg to a clinic or hospital department) for any family planning service which he or she may not give; for example, not all GPs fit diaphragms, caps or IUDs. Family planning supplies are dispensed free of charge on a prescription with the exception of condoms. Prescriptions are dispensed by a pharmacist in the majority of cases.

Domiciliary family planning

Domiciliary family planning services are provided on a small scale in the UK and involve a doctor or nurse visiting a woman at her home. Alternatively, they may accompany her to a clinic if she is unable to go to a clinic or to her GP for advice and help on birth control. A member of the primary health care team can arrange this.

Other family planning services

There are various non-NHS family planning clinics in the UK; some are private and some are charitable.

Private clinics

Private, fee-paying clinics in various parts of the country are available, such as the British Pregnancy Advisory Service and Marie Stopes House (Marie Stopes International).

Family planning organisations

The role of the UK FPA

The FPA is the leading UK voluntary organisation combining sexual health and family planning. It became a charity in 1962.

Celebrating its 60th anniversary in 1990, the FPA has a unique and outstanding reputation, based on pioneering work. The FPA's success in winning the right to family planning and contraception, thus relieving the suffering, ill health and poverty caused by frequent child-bearing, is one of the most notable contributions to family life this century.

In 1974 the FPA helped achieve the aim of free, accessible family planning for all when, together with other organisations, it persuaded the government to include family planning as part of the National Health Service. The FPA's clinics were transferred to the NHS, and a year later GPs also began providing free contraceptive services.

Since the transfer of its clinics to the NHS the FPA has shifted its focus from direct service provision. Its primary aim is:

'To promote sexual health and family planning by means of information, research, education, training, publications and publicity.'

Equality of opportunity in sexual health and family planning is vital.

The FPA recognises that needs may vary depending on gender, age, class, race, culture and mental and physical disability.

The FPA seeks to promote informed choice not only by ensuring people have accurate information, awareness and knowledge of sexual health, but also by encouraging appropriate social measures, policies and legislation.

Information and research

Information activities form an integral and vital part of all FPA work. The knowledge and feedback gained from contact with the general public and professionals serves to underpin the FPA's information, education and research work nationwide. The FPA provides a nation-wide information service on all aspects of contraception, reproductive and sexual health, including information on all services available in the UK. The information service is supported by the four UK Departments of Health through the health promotion agencies of the UK; the Health Education Authority for England, the Health Education Board for Scotland, Health Promotion Wales and the Health Promotion Agency for Northern Ireland.

The information service provides accurate, objective and authoritative information for the general public and professionals on all aspects of family planning, reproductive and sexual health through a fully established nation-wide information advice, research and consultancy service. In addition it seeks to set standards in information and advice both within the FPA and outside. The information service is provided through a centralised information and research department at National Office in London and through the FPA centres in Wales, Northern Ireland and Scotland in order that local needs are met. The FPA holds a complete and up-to-date index of all UK family planning clinic addresses and session times, as well as related reproductive help agencies. The FPA's reference library of selected journals, books, government publications and statistics, parliamentary material, topic files and press cuttings forms a unique information and research database on family planning, reproductive and sexual health.

The information service's telephone helpline is open for the public and professionals from Monday to Friday, between 10.00am and 3.00pm. The library can be visited by appointment.

The FPA's research and health policy role is now firmly established and respected. It is concerned with identifying and addressing key elements of debate linking research and raising awareness in family planning, sexual and reproductive health.

Publicity and publications

The FPA actively seeks to raise public awareness and debate around the issues relating to sexual health and family planning. Through a planned programme of media and press publicity, the FPA aims to inform and educate both the general public and professionals. The FPA press office is in constant day-to-day contact with hundreds of journalists and programme makers, providing information, comment and advice so as to ensure accurate and balanced coverage.

As part of its education and information work, the FPA produces a very wide range of publications for the general public and for professionals. This includes public information leaflets on all the family planning methods, of which over four million copies a year are distributed through health promotion units in the UK. Thoroughly consumer-tested and researched, with the latest medical information, all these publications are approved by the Plain English Campaign and carry the Crystal Mark for clarity of language and design.

In addition, the FPA has developed a unique series of training resources and books for health and other professionals. These include practical and informative reference guides, teaching manuals, factsheets and the quarterly newsletter for health professionals, *Family Planning Today*.

All FPA publications are available from the FPA's book shop, Healthwise, which also stocks over 800 other publications on family planning, sexual health, relationships and sexuality. These are available either by mail order or direct from Healthwise which is open Monday to Friday 9.00am to 5.00pm (4.30pm on Friday) at 35 Mortimer Street, London WIN 7RJ. (Write, or telephone 071 636 7866 for free catalogues.)

Education and training

The FPA's Education and Training Department provides training and consultancy to those with a professional responsibility for sexual health in health and social services and education.

The department provides training for those promoting sexual health in schools, the community, the workplace, and those working in primary and secondary care to have awareness, confidence and skills in relation to sexuality. The department works with:

▶ health authorities, to define regional and district strategies in areas of sexual health
▶ purchasers and providers of family planning and sexual health services to ensure that these are designed to meet the specific needs of local communities and run by staff with ability to communicate with a range of people about sexuality
▶ school teachers, governors and nurses on the development of appropriate and sensitive school sex education

A programme of short courses is run each year and a range of courses are designed to meet the specific training needs of sponsoring authorities and organisations.

Faculty of Family Planning and Reproductive Health Care of the Royal College of Obstetricians and Gynaecologists (RCOG)

The formation of this new RCOG Faculty in 1993 is the result of many years' work to improve and advance the speciality of family planning and improve the career structure and status of family planning doctors. The Faculty replaces NAFPD and the JCC and its main objectives are to:

▶ give academic status to the discipline of family planning and reproductive health care and recognise the expertise within it
▶ maintain and develop standards of care and training and ensure that a high quality of practice is maintained by all providers of family planning and reproductive health care
▶ promote the effective interaction of reproductive health care with related disciplines
▶ gather, collate and provide information in support of basic and continuing education in the discipline
▶ advance medical knowledge in the discipline and encourage audit and research
▶ support and represent those working in the discipline at regional, national and international levels

The Faculty will grant diplomas, certificates or equivalent recognition of specialist knowledge and skills in family planning and reproductive health care. In addition it promotes conferences and lectures, provides an advisory service and publishes the *British Journal of Family Planning.*

National Association of Family Planning Doctors (NAFPD)

In 1974 the service role of the FPA was largely taken over by the NHS. Until then doctors and nurses working within family planning services had been members of the medical and nursing bodies of the FPA. The National Association of Family Planning Doctors (NAFPD) was set up in 1974 to provide an organisation for doctors with an interest in or working in the area of family planning. It has now been replaced by the Faculty of Family Planning and Reproductive Health Care.

Joint Committee on Contraception (JCC)

Set up in 1974 by the FPA, NAFPD and the RCOG, the JCC was the body responsible for training in family planning and certification of doctors and instructing doctors. This function has now been incorporated into the Faculty of Family Planning and Reproductive Health Care.

National Association of Family Planning Nurses (NAFPN)

Membership to NAFPN is open to all registered nurses, midwives and health visitors who hold a recognised family planning qualification. It aims to facilitate study and the exchange of information and to promote training in family planning.

Royal College of Nursing (RCN) Family Planning Forum

This is one of a number of special interest groups of the RCN. Its main objectives are to:

▶ establish a corporate identity for RCN members engaged in the speciality of family planning nursing
▶ increase knowledge and skills in family planning
▶ act as a resource to the RCN

Family planning and the pharmacist

Pharmacists have a huge fund of knowledge that is highly valuable to family planning and health professionals. Pharmacists often receive more direct feedback from patients than other health professionals especially about such factors as compliance and palatability of medicines. Pharmacists often see people with initial concerns or worries and are therefore in a good position to refer.

Importantly pharmacists today are fully involved in the wider role of health promotion in the everyday setting of a pharmacy or hospital. Pharmacists can advise and supply certain contraceptive methods that do not require a prescription as well as dispensing contraception on prescription. They are therefore in constant contact with people who may seek advice about contraception and related areas. Because pharmacists are not authoritarian medical figures and are easily accessible in pharmacies, they have an invaluable role in providing information about family planning and sexual health and in enabling women and men to effectively seek further help from health and medical professionals. The pharmacist's knowledge of medical matters, and specifically of drugs and drug interactions make them an important part of the health care team today.

Conception

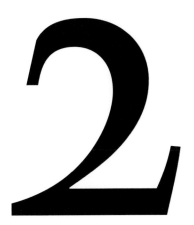

The male

Sperm production

Sperm are produced in the seminiferous tubules within the testes. They then move into the epididymis where they mature and develop. From production to maturity takes about three months and is a continual process. Mature sperm pass through the vas deferens to be stored in the seminal vesicles near the prostate gland. When a man is sexually excited and has an erection, the stored sperm enter the urethra where secretions from the prostate are added. This fluid is the semen and it is expelled by muscular contractions of the penis when the man ejaculates.

The female

Ovulation

A woman's menstrual cycle begins with the onset of the menstrual period. This cycle is controlled by the pituitary hormones – follicle stimulating hormone (FSH) and luteinising hormone (LH), and the ovarian hormones – oestrogen and progestogen. The pituitary hormones trigger follicle development where one of the eggs within the ovary matures and, about 12-16 days *before* the beginning of her next period, the mature egg is released from the ovary. The egg enters the funnel-shaped end of the fallopian tube and is transported down the fallopian tube by contractions of the tube and by movement of cilia lining the tube.

Passage of sperm/cervical mucus

Once in the woman's vagina, the sperm enter the womb through the cervix by passing through the cervical mucus. When the woman is in the fertile period of her menstrual cycle (around ovulation) fertile cervical mucus is produced which is thin and slippery and allows the sperm to pass into the womb where they swim up to the fallopian tubes. At other times in the cycle, the cervical mucus – non-fertile mucus – is less easily penetrated and acts as a barrier to sperm entering the womb.

Fertilisation

Fertilisation usually takes place in the fallopian tube. The fertilised egg then travels down to the womb, where under the influence of oestrogen the lining has thickened ready to receive it. The fertilised egg, dividing all the time, begins to implant in the endometrium about five to seven days after ovulation.

Implantation

The implanted early embryo produces a hormone, human chorionic gonadotrophin (hCG), which enters the blood-stream and reaches the ovary where it acts to maintain the corpus luteum. The corpus luteum produces the hormone progesterone which sustains the pregnancy. Not all eggs that are released are fertilised, and of those that are, many do not implant, or fail to develop properly and are rejected.

Contraception

3

**General
introduction**

Contraception involves an interruption in the normal physiological events leading to conception. This is achieved by control of ovulation or by using methods that prevent fertilisation by stopping the egg and the sperm meeting. There are many methods available.

**Unreliable
methods and
popular
fallacies**

There is some truth in the statement that any method is better than none. Probably the most commonly used (but not well documented) is coitus interruptus or 'withdrawal' (often described as 'being careful'). This method is unreliable because ejaculation is difficult to control and some sperm may be released before the penis is withdrawn. Those using this method should be given information about more reliable alternatives. No-one however should be discouraged from using any method if it works for them and they choose not to use another.

Myths

There are many myths in circulation about contraception which are inaccurate. Whatever people say, the facts are that:

▶ breast-feeding does not always prevent pregnancy
▶ pregnancy can occur if the woman does not have an orgasm, and intercourse in any position can result in pregnancy
▶ pregnancy can follow the first intercourse, can occur without full penetration, and occasionally results when intercourse takes place during the woman's period
▶ douching is useless as a contraceptive measure and persistent douching may damage the vaginal mucosa and cause other problems

Many people are not sure how their bodies work and may need help in understanding contraception. Health professionals are in an ideal position to provide accurate information and help.

Methods available

Regular methods

▶ combined oral contraceptive (COC)

▶ contraceptive implants

▶ progestogen-only pill (POP)

▶ injectable contraception

▶ intrauterine contraceptive device (IUDs)

▶ female barrier methods: diaphragm or cap and spermicide, and female condoms

▶ spermicides and the vaginal contraceptive sponge

▶ male condoms

▶ natural family planning

▶ male and female sterilisation

Effectiveness of contraceptive methods

See Table 1 for the efficacy of the different methods.

Emergency methods

Postcoital contraception:

▶ hormonal method

▶ IUD method

The FPA produces leaflets for the general public on all the methods of family planning.

Data about the efficacy of methods vary, it is important to recognise the difference between *method-failures* – ie pregnancies occurring despite the method being used absolutely correctly during every act of intercourse and *user-failures* – where pregnancy has occurred due to incorrect use or non-use of a method on one or more occasions. Method-effectiveness rates vary because of physiological differences between individuals and aspects such as age. User effectiveness is related to the motivation of the individual, which is strongly dependent on how contraception is discussed and how contraceptive services are delivered.

Where contraceptives work

Female

1 Combined pill
prevents ovulation

2 IUD
prevents sperm reaching the egg

3 Injectables
prevents ovulation
Implants
effect on cervix and ovulation

4 Sterilisation
stops egg reaching the womb

5 Diaphragm and cap + spermicide, sponge, female condom
prevents sperm reaching the egg

6 Progestogen-only pill
effect mainly on cervix

Natural methods
find 'safest' day to avoid pregnancy

Male

1 Vasectomy
stops sperm release

2 Male condom
prevents sperm reaching the egg

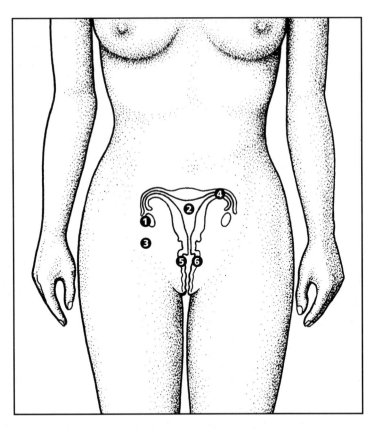

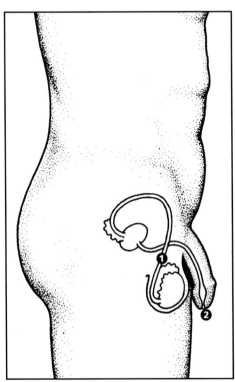

Table 1 User efficacy of available contraceptive methods

	% per 100 women per year
Sterilisation	Occasional failures occur (1 in 1,000 male sterilisations) (1-3 per 1,000 female sterilisations)
Contraceptive implant	99-almost 100% effective
Injectable contraceptive	Almost 100% effective
Combined oral contraceptive	97-almost 100% effective with careful use
Progestogen-only pill	96-99% effective with careful use*
Intrauterine device	98-almost 100% effective
Condoms (male and female)	85-98% effective with careful use
Diaphragm or cap + spermicide	85-98% effective with careful use
Vaginal contraceptive sponge	75-91% effective with careful use
Natural family planning (sympto-thermal method)	80-98% effective with careful use

* **Note:** Research suggests that the efficacy of progestogen-only pills may be reduced in some women weighing over 70 kg (11 stones).

Oral contraceptives

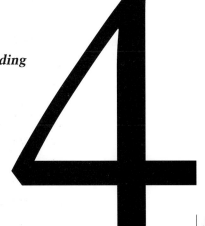

Combined oral contraceptives

General information

The combined oral contraceptive pill is one of the most effective reversible methods of contraception. If the pill is taken consistently, according to instructions, the chance of pregnancy occurring is practically nil. All oral contraceptives are medicinal products and they are supplied only on a doctor's prescription. The pill should be taken only after discussion and medical examination to exclude possible contraindications and the woman should return for regular check-ups.

Mode of action

Combined oral contraceptives contain synthetic oestrogen and progestogen. They prevent ovulation by suppressing the secretion of gonadotrophins by the hypothalamus and pituitary. In addition these pills prevent changes in the endometrium which are usually needed for pregnancy implantation; they inhibit spermatozoal transport through altered cervical mucus and interfere with normal mobility and secretion in the fallopian tubes.

Efficacy

Theoretically the pill is an extremely effective reversible method of contraception when it is taken correctly and consistently, is absorbed normally, and its metabolism is not affected by interaction with other medication. In practice, its use effectiveness varies and pregnancy rates range from 0.1-3 per cent (the latter figure can be higher and reflects poor usage).

Preparations available

See *British National Formulary* (section 7.3.1) and *MIMS* and Tables 2 and 3 on pages 48 and 49. The combined oral contraceptives available in the UK contain synthetic oestrogen (either ethinyloestradiol or mestranol) and a progestogen (levonorgestrel, norgestrel, ethynodiol diacetate, norethisterone, norethisterone acetate, desogestrel, gestodene or norgestimate). The name levonorgestrel formerly known as D-norgestrel refers to the active isomer of the progestogen norgestrel.

The most widely used preparations contain 30 to 40 micrograms of oestrogen or less. Occasionally preparations containing 50 micrograms of oestrogen are prescribed. No contraceptive preparations available in the UK contain more than 50 micrograms of oestrogen.

Dose

In order to minimise any possible long-term adverse effect, the recommendation from the FPA and the National Association of Family Planning Doctors (NAFPD) – now the Faculty of Family Planning and Reproductive Health Care – is that the pill of choice should be the one containing the lowest *acceptable* dose of oestrogen and progestogen which:

▶ provides effective contraception
▶ produces good menstrual cycle control
▶ is associated with fewest side-effects ·
▶ has the least known effect on carbohydrate and lipid metabolism and metabolic parameters

Types of combined pills

Monophasic pills

Monophasic pills are the most widely used combined pills and come in packets of 21 identical tablets which are taken on 21 consecutive days. The pills are then stopped for 7 days during which some withdrawal bleeding will usually occur. After 7 pill-free days the next packet of pills is started. This routine is continued as long as contraception is required.

Phasic pills – biphasic and triphasic types

The hormone content of phasic pills varies throughout the cycle. They aim to provide a lower total dose of hormone over each cycle. The different strengths of pill must be taken in the right order for 21 days, as marked on the packet, followed by 7 pill-free days.

Everyday (ED) pills

Everyday combined pills (ED pills) are available for those who find it easier to take pills every day without a break. Of the 28 pills, seven are inactive, so need to be taken in the right order. There are monophasic and triphasic varieties of ED pills.

Advantages

▶ one of the most reliable, reversible, convenient, non-intercourse related methods
▶ often relieves painful periods (dysmenorrhoea) and may make bleeding lighter and more regular
▶ decreases the risk of iron deficiency anaemia
▶ often relieves premenstrual symptoms
▶ reduces the risk of benign breast disease
▶ reduces the risk of fibroids and ovarian cysts
▶ protects against endometrial and ovarian cancer
▶ protects against pelvic inflammatory disease (PID)
▶ reduction in the rate of endometriosis

Disadvantages

▶ effectiveness depends on comprehensive instruction and correct usage
▶ unsuitable for women with contraindications or risk factors for circulatory problems
▶ possible minor side-effects when first starting the pill, such as headaches, weight gain, breakthrough bleeding
▶ increased incidence of some problems in some women, such as hypertension, arterial and venous disease
▶ not suitable for smokers over the age of 35
▶ problems with potential drug interactions
▶ uncertainties about the combined pill and breast and cervical cancer (see page 42)
▶ no protection against STDs, including HIV

Absolute contra-indications

For *full* information see Manufacturer's data sheet.

▶ possible pregnancy
▶ abnormal vaginal or uterine bleeding of unknown cause
▶ cardiovascular disease, or risk factors for
▶ past history of thrombosis of any type
▶ disorders of lipid metabolism
▶ focal or crescendo migraine or migraine requiring ergotamine treatment
▶ markedly impaired liver function

▶ known or suspected malignancy of the breast, liver or genital tract

▶ past pruritus, Pemphigus gestationis, deteriorating otosclerotic deafness, or unexplained jaundice during early pregnancy

▶ recent trophoblastic disease and elevated hCG levels

▶ gall bladder disease

▶ psychosis or severe depression

▶ four weeks before major or leg surgery

▶ ulcerative colitis (UC) or Crohn's with severe attacks

The pill should only be given with special care to women who have, or have had, diabetes mellitus, elevated blood pressure, conditions such as epilepsy, obesity, cardiac or renal dysfunction, sickle cell anaemia, fibroids, or to smokers over 35.

Instructions for use of combined pills

Monophasic pills 21-day pill

Many preparations are available with a variety of progestogens and oestrogens in different doses. The first packet is usually started on day 1 of the period without using an additional contraceptive method, (or less commonly, up to day 5 of the menstrual cycle using an additional method for the first 7 days).

Phasic combined pills (biphasic and triphasic) 21-day pill

The first packet is started on day 1 of the period without the need for an additional contraceptive method, or up to day 5 of the menstrual cycle using an additional contraceptive method for the first 7 days. The pills must be taken in the correct order.

ED combined pills 28-day pill (monophasic or triphasic)

The first packet is started on day 1 of the period. Additional contraceptive precautions must be used for the first 14 days. This is because the start day may occur with inactive not active pills. The pills must be taken every day in the correct order.

Missed pills

Ideally, oral contraceptives should be taken at a regular time each day, as their efficacy can fall if they are taken late or omitted. A combined pill is regarded as 'missed' if it is taken more than 12 hours late. If it is remembered within 12 hours, contraceptive protection is not lost. If it is taken more than 12 hours late contraceptive protection is lost. The missed pill should be taken as soon as it is remembered. The next pill should be taken at the normal time. This may mean more than one pill is taken in one day. If more than one pill is missed, the last missed pill should be taken and the rest of the packet taken at the normal time. An extra contraceptive method must be used for 7 days. Where there are less than 7 days' worth of pills in the pack, the pack should be finished, and a new packet should be started immediately and continued *without* a break. With ED pills, if the 7 days run into the end of the packet, the 7 inactive pills should be missed out and the next packet started immediately without any break.

These guidelines now are the accepted standardised guidelines for missed pill advice, and have been *agreed* by the major oral contraceptive manufacturers and the main family planning organisations in the UK.

Periods

Most women who do not take the pill have normal menstrual cycles varying from 21 to 42 days. While taking combined pills this pattern is replaced by regular withdrawal bleeds which follow 48-72 hours after discontinuing the last *active* pill. These 'periods' are usually lighter and shorter on the combined pill. Withdrawal bleeds can be postponed for special occasions or travel and pill-taking can be adjusted. The instructions for this vary with different pills. To miss a withdrawal bleed on monophasic pills, the pills should be continued without a break (with ED pills – the inactive pills are omitted). Phasic pills are more complex, but the principal is to continue with the same or equivalent dose of progestogen to prevent a drop in hormone level. The advice here is to use the last phase of a 'spare' packet which will give 7, 10 or 14 days postponement (depending on brand) of the withdrawal bleed. Women should be advised that in some cases breakthrough bleeding may occur.

Breakthrough or irregular bleeding

Spotting or irregular bleeding is common in the first few cycles of starting the pill. If this persists beyond 3 months a change of pill is indicated. Women should be warned of this possibility and advised to *continue* the pill-taking as normal, whether bleeding or not.

Bleeding in a pill taker can also be due to the following reasons, which should be considered when giving advice:

► default, ie missing pills
► very severe diarrhoea and/or vomiting
► drugs which interact
► diet (reported in a few vegetarians/vegans)
► disease (especially of cervix or in pregnancy)
► dose of preparation being used

Any irregular bleeding should *always* be investigated.

Missed period

If a period is missed, and the pill has been taken regularly and correctly, it is unlikely that pregnancy is the cause. If a withdrawal bleed has not occurred the possibility of pregnancy should be excluded before the next packet of pills is started. This is often not practical; if the next packet is not started and if alternative contraception is not used there could be a risk of unplanned pregnancy. However if *two* withdrawal bleeds have been missed, the next packet of pills should not be started until the possibility of pregnancy has been excluded. Pregnancy tests today allow for early diagnosis of pregnancy. Taking oral contraceptives does not alter pregnancy test results.

Smoking
It is not advisable for women taking oral contraceptives to smoke. It may be helpful to give smokers suitable literature eg *So you want to stop smoking*, a booklet

produced by the Health Education Authority. Heavy smokers (defined as those smoking 20 or more cigarettes a day) may be refused the combined pill until they have given up smoking.

Stomach upsets

Vomiting within three hours of taking the pill, or very severe diarrhoea can interfere with the absorption of the pill. Women seeking simple remedies for these symptoms while on the pill should be reminded to use additional contraceptive precautions (eg a condom), for *any intercourse* during the illness, and for 7 days after recovery (see 'Instructions for use of combined pills' on page 37).

Changing pills

When changing from a higher dose preparation to a lower dose preparation, or from a combined pill to a progestogen-only pill, or vice versa, the first pill of the new packet should be taken on the next day immediately after the old packet is completed. No extra contraceptive method is necessary.

Planning a pregnancy

A woman planning a baby should stop taking the pill at the end of the packet. Ideally it is best to wait for one natural period using another method of contraception, before trying to become pregnant. This allows the body to return to its 'pre-pill' state, allowing the pregnancy to be dated more accurately and to allow for good 'pre-pregnancy' care. Should conception occur before this time, there is no evidence of increased birth defects, or problems with pregnancy.

Using the pill after childbirth

Following childbirth, combined pills can be started at any time after 3 weeks postpartum (not earlier because of the increased risk of thrombosis in relation to the combined pill, and of breakthrough bleeding in relation to the progestogen-only pill). If the combined pill is started later than 3 weeks postpartum, an extra contraceptive method should be used for the first 7 days.

Breast-feeding

Women who are breast-feeding should avoid oestrogen-containing pills. Oestrogen affects lactation. Progestogen-only pills are suitable, if a hormonal method is wanted.

Using the pill after an abortion or miscarriage

The combined pill can be started immediately after a first or second trimester miscarriage or abortion, as it does not interfere with recovery or increase morbidity.

Operations/ surgery

Combined pills which contain oestrogen should be discontinued (and adequate contraceptive arrangements made) 4 weeks before major elective surgery and all surgery to the legs; they should normally be restarted on the first period occurring at least 2 weeks after mobilisation after the operation. When discontinuation is not possible, eg after trauma or if a patient admitted for an elective procedure is by oversight still on an oestrogen-containing oral contraceptive, some consideration should be given to subcutaneous heparin prophylaxis. These recommendations do not apply to minor surgery, eg tooth extractions, laparoscopy.

Using the pill after unprotected intercourse

Special doses of the pill can be used as a postcoital method within 72 hours of unprotected intercourse (see 'Emergency Contraception' on page 115).

Duration of use

There is no medical evidence for routine 'breaks' in pill use. It is worth remembering that a woman has 13 breaks, each lasting a week, every single year. Use of the pill has not been linked to infertility. A healthy non-smoking woman with no medical contraindications can use the combined pill until the menopause.

Side-effects

Women may initially experience slight nausea, headaches, depression, breast swelling, breast tenderness, tiredness, weight increase or changes in libido. Intolerance to contact lenses may develop. Irregular (breakthrough) bleeding may occur, especially in the first month or two. These symptoms may disappear spontaneously if women are reassured and encouraged to persevere (see 'Breakthrough or irregular bleeding' on page 39).

Side-effects that persist should always be investigated.

Risks

The more serious side-effects, such as thrombosis or strokes are uncommon but the risks are greater in women with diabetes and those whose close relatives have had heart attacks or strokes at an early age (under 45), those with over-weight problems, elevated blood pressure and those who smoke. These risks increase with age and for this reason, women smokers over 35 will be discouraged from taking the combined oral contraceptive pill. Women taking the pill should in general be encouraged to stop smoking.

Oral contraceptives and breast and cervical cancer

The literature on this is complex and contradictory at present. Some studies have suggested a possible association between the use of oral contraceptives and the risk of developing breast cancer under the age of 35 or so (several years of combined pill use at an early age before a full first term pregnancy) or cervical cancer. Other studies fail to show the same association. Due to such conflicting research a number of studies are under way to provide a clearer picture.

The incidence of breast cancer is high in women living in the UK. It must therefore be expected to develop in women whether they take oral contraceptives or not. In the UK the lifetime risk is between one in 12 and one in 14. Risk factors include: genetic predisposition (breast cancer in mother or sister), early menarche, late menopause, nulliparity, benign breast disease, high fat diet, post-menopausal use of unopposed oestrogen and being aged over 40. Protective factors include: early first pregnancy, early oophorectomy, lactation and early menopause.

With regard to cervical cancer, sexual behaviour (age at first intercourse, number of sexual partners), multiple pregnancies, cigarette smoking, sexually transmitted infections and socio-economic status are important determinants of cancer of the cervix.

Such determinants associated with breast and cervical cancer make it difficult to be precise about the role of oral contraceptive use and the risk of these two cancers.

Advice from the Committee on the Safety of Medicines

The Committee on the Safety of Medicines (CSM) has stated that it is important to balance the uncertainties in relation to carcinoma of the breast and cervix against the evidence available that combined oral contraceptives protect against ovarian and endometrial carcinoma. Taking into account both the benefits and potential risks of oral contraceptive use, the CSM recommends that there is no need for a change in oral contraceptive prescribing practice on the evidence presently available.

Other symptoms   Although women should be aware of the risks of the pill, it must be emphasised that the number of women who actually encounter problems is extremely small, and for most women the benefits of the pill outweigh the possible disadvantages.

For a fuller review of side-effects see 'Recommended reading' on pages 160-162.

Women should be investigated immediately if they develop any of the following:

▶ painful swelling of a calf
▶ pain in the chest or abdomen
▶ breathlessness or cough with blood-stained phlegm
▶ a bad fainting attack or collapse
▶ unusual headache or disturbance of speech or eyesight
▶ numbness or weakness of a limb
▶ jaundice (yellow skin or yellow eyes)
▶ severe and generalised skin rash

Although not pill-related, symptoms such as lumps in the breast, discharge from a nipple, or bleeding after sexual intercourse should be investigated promptly.

Drugs and combined oral contraceptives

Oral contraceptive efficacy may in some instances be reduced by concurrent drug taking, and oral contraceptives may sometimes modify the action of a particular drug being taken. This section will only address drugs and reduced oral contraceptive efficacy.

Certain drugs are known to reduce the efficacy of oral contraceptives in some women. Pregnancies have occurred as a result of interactions between oral contraceptives and antibacterials as well as anticonvulsant drugs and certain analgesics, sedatives and tranquillisers. Although the evidence for reduced efficacy of oral contraceptives with broad spectrum antibiotics is based on small numbers, it is prudent to recommend additional contraceptive cover for women taking certain antibiotics and oral contraceptives. It is particularly important to advise an extra contraceptive method when enzyme inducers, especially rifampicin, griseofulvin, and most anticonvulsants are taken as these significantly reduce blood concentrations of both oestrogen and progestogen.

The main drugs which may reduce the efficacy of combined oral contraceptives

Anticonvulsant drugs and barbiturates

Many common anticonvulsants induce hepatic drug metabolising enzymes thereby lowering levels of both oestrogen and progestogen. The newly introduced drugs such as vigabatrin, lamotrigine and clobazam do not have this property and neither do older drugs such as sodium valproate and clonazepam.

A number of pregnancies have been reported in women receiving combined oral contraceptives and:

▶ Phenobarbitone
▶ Hydantoins (phenytoin)
▶ Primidone
▶ Carbamazepine

Barbiturates, and to a lesser extent, hydantoins and primidone are microsomal enzyme inducers in humans, and may increase the rate of metabolism of contraceptive steroids.

Advice

A higher dose of ethinyloestradiol containing 50 micrograms or more is advisable if alternative methods of contraception are inappropriate for women with epilepsy. It is also suggested that the recommendation of 'tricycling' using monophasic pills is useful for some women. This involves taking three of four packets in a row followed by a short tablet-free interval of 4 days. This reduces the number of pill free episodes. Caution is advised when enzyme inducers are withdrawn, since it takes some time for the liver's level of excretory function to revert to normal. So advice needs to be taken on how long extra contraceptive cover is required after drug therapy. Medical opinion suggests 4 to 8 weeks of extra contraceptive cover is required depending on which enzyme inducer has been used.

Antituberculous drugs

Rifampicin is a potent enzyme inducing drug. The majority of women who use oral contraceptives concurrently with rifampicin have poor cycle control (ie irregular bleeding) and a number of pregnancies have been reported. Therefore it is normal practice to *always* advise an alternative method of contraception. Short term use of rifampicin (ie a short course to clear meningococci from the nose) also requires additional contraceptive precautions over this time *and* for 4 weeks after.

Antibacterials/antifungals

A small number of pregnancies have occurred in women taking combined oral contraceptives and

antibacterials:

- ▶ Ampicillin
- ▶ Amoxycillin
- ▶ Augmentin
- ▶ Erythromycin
- ▶ Tetracyclines
- ▶ Cephalosporins
- ▶ Rifampicin (see antituberculous drugs and information on enzyme inducers)

antifungals:

- ▶ Griseofulvin (see information on enzyme inducers)

Antibiotic-induced changes in gut bacteria may affect the enterohepatic circulation of ethinyloestradiol and reduce plasma levels.

Advice

Broad spectrum antibiotics interact only with oestrogen (so the progestogen-only pill is unaffected). Certain antibiotics alter the colonic flora and reduce their capacity to hydrolyse oestrogen conjugates in the enterophepatic circulation back into active oestrogen. If such an antibiotic is continued for 2 weeks or so, the flora develop resistance and oestrogen levels rise back to normal. Thus women on long-term antibiotics, eg for acne, need not take extra contraceptive precautions.

The FPA recommends that women on oral contraceptives should use additional contraceptive cover during a short course (two weeks or less) of antibiotics, and for 7 days after the last antibiotic tablet. If the 7 days run beyond the end of a packet then a new packet should be started immediately and continued without a break. With ED pills the inactive pills should be missed out (see 'Instructions for use of combined pills' on page 37).

Analgesics

Oral contraceptive efficacy can possibly be reduced with analgesics containing phenacetin or pyrazolones.

Sedatives and tranquillisers

Pregnancies have rarely been reported in women receiving oral contraceptives and:

▶ Diazepam (large doses intravenously)
▶ Chlorpromazine
▶ Chlordiazepoxide

Recreational drugs

Breakthrough bleeding has been reported while using combined oral contraceptive pills and recreational drugs. There is however, no pharmacological basis for an interaction between the two. The irregular bleeding is most likely due to default in pill taking.

Vitamins

There is no reduction in the efficiency of combined oral contraceptives and vitamins. However, it should be noted that megadoses of ascorbic acid (vitamin C) of 0.5-1g daily convert a low dose oestrogen pill into a high dose pill. This is due to competition for sulphate conjugation in the bowel wall. On discontinuing vitamin C, breakthrough bleeding may occur.

For a full review of drugs and oral contraceptives see British National Formulary and 'Recommended reading' on page 160.

Anti-androgen pills

Dianette

Dianette is an anti-androgen/oestrogen combination for the oral treatment of acne, seborrhoea and mild hirsutism in women which is also a reliable contraceptive. Dianette contains 2mg cyproterone acetate and 35mcg ethinyl-oestradiol in packs of 21 tablets. It is not primarily prescribed for contraception.

General follow-up

Women should be seen as instructed, this is usually every six months. Where a prescription is written for 13 months, a woman should be seen where possible after at least six months.

Women should *always* be encouraged to ask their family doctor or clinic if there are any worries or concerns about any aspect of pill-taking.

Table 2 Monophasic combined oral contraceptives

Pill type & preparation	Manufacturer	Oestrogen (mcg)	Progestogen (mg)	
Combined – monophasic				
Ethinyloestradiol/norethisterone type				
Loestrin 20	Parke-Davis	20	1	norethisterone acetate*
Loestrin 30	Parke-Davis	30	1.5	norethisterone acetate*
Conova 30	Gold Cross	30	2	ethynodiol diacetate*
Brevinor	Syntex	35	0.5	norethisterone
Ovysmen	Ortho (Cilag)	35	0.5	norethisterone
Neocon 1/35	Ortho (Cilag)	35	1	norethisterone
Norimin	Syntex	35	1	norethisterone
Ethinyloestradiol/levonorgestrel				
Microgynon 30	Schering	30	0.15	
Ovranette	Wyeth	30	0.15	
Eugynon 30	Schering	30	0.25	
Ovran 30	Wyeth	30	0.25	
Ovran	Wyeth	50	0.25	
Ethinyloestradiol/desogestrel				
Mercilon	Organon	20	0.15	
Marvelon	Organon	30	0.15	
Ethinyloestradiol/gestodene				
Femodene (also ED)	Schering	30	0.075	
Minulet	Wyeth	30	0.075	
Ethinyloestradiol/norgestimate				
Cilest	Ortho (Cilag)	35	0.25	
Mestranol/norethisterone				
Norinyl-1	Syntex	50	1	
Ortho-Novin 1/50	Ortho (Cilag)	50	1	

* Converted (> 90%) to norethisterone as the active metabolite
Reproduced with permission of MIMS 1993

Table 3 Phasic combined oral contraceptives

Pill type & preparation	Manufacturer	Oestrogen (mcg)	Progestogen (mg)	
Biphasic & Triphasic				
Ethinyloestradiol / norethisterone				
BiNovum	Ortho (Cilag)	35	0.5	(7 tabs)
		35	1	(14 tabs)
Synphase	Syntex	35	0.5	(7 tabs)
		35	1	(9 tabs)
		35	0.5	(5 tabs)
TriNovum (also ED)	Ortho (Cilag)	35	0.5	(7 tabs)
		35	0.75	(7 tabs)
		35	1	(7 tabs)
Ethinyloestradiol / levonorgestrel				
Logynon (also ED)	Schering	30	0.05	(6 tabs)
		40	0.075	(5 tabs)
		30	0.125	(10 tabs)
Trinordiol	Wyeth	30	0.05	(6 tabs)
		40	0.075	(5 tabs)
		30	0.125	(10 tabs)
Ethinyloestradiol / gestodene				
Tri-Minulet	Wyeth	30	0.05	(6 tabs)
		40	0.07	(5 tabs)
		30	0.1	(10 tabs)
Triadene	Schering	30	0.05	(6 tabs)
		40	0.07	(5 tabs)
		30	0.1	(10 tabs)

Reproduced with permission of MIMS 1993

Progestogen-only pills

General information

Progestogen-only pills (POP) contain no oestrogen. They contain progestogen only. They are a useful alternative for women wishing to use oral contraception who choose not to use oestrogen or where oestrogens are contraindicated, such as women over 35 years who smoke and breast-feeding mothers.

Mode of action

The progestogen-only pill does not always prevent ovulation. (It prevents ovulation in 15-40 per cent of cycles). Progestogen acts on the cervical mucus, endometrium and fallopian tubes, causing changes that make it difficult for sperm to enter the womb, and rendering the lining of the womb unreceptive to the egg if fertilised.

Efficacy

The progestogen-only pill, contrary to public opinion, is a very effective method of contraception when taken correctly and consistently. In practice, its use effectiveness varies and pregnancy rates range from 1-4 per cent. Some research suggests that the efficacy rate of progestogen-only methods is reduced in some women weighing over 70kg (11 stones).

Preparations available

See *British National Formulary* (section 7.3.2) and *MIMS* and Table 4.

Progestogen-only pills contain low doses of the following progestogens: norethisterone, ethynodiol diacetate (converts to norethisterone) or levonorgestrel.

Advantages

▶ easy and convenient to use
▶ non-intercourse related method
▶ suitable for older women who smoke and those who are breast-feeding
▶ suitable for women who cannot use oestrogen containing oral contraceptives
▶ may relieve premenstrual tension and dysmenorrhoea
▶ minimal alteration in carbohydrate and lipid metabolism

▶ no evidence of increased risk of cardiovascular disease, thromboembolism or hypertension

Disadvantages
▶ not as effective as combined pills
▶ must be taken at a regular time to achieve optimum effectiveness
▶ disruption of menstrual pattern
▶ increased spotting or breakthrough bleeding
▶ possible increase in ectopic pregnancy in the event of POP failure
▶ a small number of women will develop functional ovarian cysts

Contra-indications

For *full* information see manufacturer's data sheet.

▶ possible pregnancy
▶ abnormal vaginal or uterine bleeding of unknown cause
▶ previous ectopic pregnancy
▶ recent trophoblastic and elevated hCG levels
▶ any known malignancy disease of the breast
▶ active liver disease, liver adenoma or carcinoma
▶ recurrent cholestatic jaundice
▶ history of jaundice in pregnancy (relative contraindication)
▶ past severe actual arterial disease or severely abnormal lipid profile
▶ any serious side-effects from use of combined oral contraceptives which were not attributed to oestrogen
▶ past hospitalisation for functional ovarian cysts
▶ unacceptability of irregular menstrual bleeding

Instructions for use of progestogen-only pills

The first packet is started on day 1 of the period without the need for additional contraceptive cover and then taken daily, without a break, even through the period.

It is important that the pill is taken at the same time each day as the efficiency falls markedly if tablets are taken late or omitted. A progestogen-only pill is regarded as 'missed' if taken only three hours late. In such cases, the missed pill should be taken immediately and normal pill taking resumed when the next pill is due. Additional contraceptive precautions should be taken for 7 days. Prior to 1993, the guideline for additional contraceptive precautions was 48 hours. This change allows for standardisation of guidelines between combined oral contraceptives and progestogen-only contraception. It should be noted that although the new 7-day advice increases concensus and consistency it does not add any important additional efficacy to the previous 2-day recommendation. The main family planning organisations and the contraceptive manufacturers are currently working together to produce common agreed guidelines on all methods of contraception based on current research and informed opinion, in order that consumers receive standardised information.

Periods

Changes in the menstrual cycle are quite common in progestogen-only pill users. Menstrual irregularity is the main problem with progestogen-only methods. This sometimes settles down after a few cycles. Spotting and breakthrough bleeding also occur in some women. For some, periods stop completely. Providing pregnancy is excluded this problem is not harmful and implies that ovulation is being inhibited. If such changes are not acceptable, a change of pill is usually indicated.

Smoking

Although it is not advisable for any women to smoke, smoking is not a contraindication to progestogen-only pills.

Stomach upsets

Vomiting within three hours of taking the pill, or very severe diarrhoea can interfere with absorption of the pill. Additional contraceptive precautions should be used over the time of illness and for 7 days after recovery. (See 'Instructions for use of progestogen-only pills' on page 51).

Changing pills

When changing from one progestogen-only pill to another, or from a combined oral contraceptive pill to a progestogen-only pill, or vice versa, the first pill of the new pack should be started on the next day immediately after the old packet is complete. No extra contraceptive method is necessary.

Planning a pregnancy	A woman planning a baby should stop taking the pill at the end of the packet. Ideally it is best to wait for one natural period using another method of contraception, before trying to become pregnant. This allows the body to return to its 'pre-pill' state, allowing the pregnancy to be dated more accurately and to allow for good 'pre-pregnancy' care. Should conception occur before this time, there is no evidence of increased birth defects, or problems with pregnancy.
After childbirth and breast-feeding	Progestogen-only pills can be taken from day 21 after birth. Taken before this time causes an increase in irregular bleeding. This pill is not contraindicated for breast-feeding mothers. Most studies have failed to demonstrate any alteration in the quality or quantity of milk. Although a small amount of progestogen may be ingested by the baby, extensive research shows no evidence of any deleterious effects.
Operations/ surgery	Progestogen-only preparations need not be discontinued if surgery is needed.
Side-effects	The main side-effect of progestogen-only pills is menstrual irregularity (see 'Periods' on page 52). Other effects include, weight gain, breast tenderness, decreased libido, acne and headaches in some women. These symptoms usually settle down after the first few cycles.
Risks	The proportion of ectopic pregnancies (ie where the pregnancy develops outside the uterus, usually in the fallopian tube), is increased in progestogen-only pill users, but the incidence is low, less than would be expected in women using no contraception. This increased risk is due to the fact that progestogen-only pills are more effective at limiting intra rather than extrauterine pregnancies. The possibility of ectopic pregnancy must always be considered in any woman who develops sudden lower abdominal pain, with light, scanty or a missed period. Women using progestogen-only methods also have increased risk of functional ovarian cysts. These may

cause pain, or may not cause any problems. They are not dangerous and do not require surgery. These cysts usually disappear.

Drug interactions with progestogen-only contraceptives

See advice on page 44 for combined oral contraceptives. However, it is important to note that there is *no* interaction between antibiotics and progestogen-only pills.

Table 4 Progestogen-only oral contraceptives

Pill type & preparation	Manufacturer	Progestogen (mg)	
Norethisterone type			
Micronor	Ortho (Cilag)	0.35	norethisterone
Noriday	Syntex	0.35	norethisterone
Femulen	Gold Cross	0.5	ethynodiol diacetate*
Levonorgestrel			
Microval	Wyeth	0.03	
Norgeston	Schering	0.03	
Neogest	Schering	0.075	norgestrel

* Converted (> 90%) to norethisterone as the active metabolite
Reproduced with permission of MIMS 1993

Injectable contraception

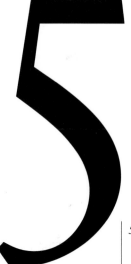

General information

There are two injectable contraceptive methods in the UK: Depo-Provera (medroxyprogesterone acetate) and Noristerat (norethisterone oenanthate).

Mode of action

Injectables work in a similar way to the progestogen-only pill, but in addition always inhibit ovulation. Both injectable preparations are given as deep intramuscular injection within the first 5 days of menstruation. Depo-Provera is given every 12 weeks and Noristerat is repeated once after 8 weeks.

Effectiveness

Both Depo-Provera and Noristerat are highly effective methods of contraception. A main advantage being no 'user' failures. The efficacy rate is 99 to almost 100 per cent.

Table 5 Injectable contraceptive products

Product & manufacturer	Chemical constituents	Dosage	Presentation
Depo-Provera (150 mg/ml) Upjohn Ltd	medroxyprogesterone acetate	A single injection of 150mg i.m. every 12 weeks	A sterile aqueous suspension of medroxyprogesterone acetate: 150 mg/ml suspended in vial 1 ml
Noristerat Schering Healthcare	norethisterone oenanthate	A single injection of 200mg i.m. repeated once after 8 weeks	200 mg/ml in a vehicle of benzyl benzoate and castor oil in 1 ml ampoules

Licensing in the UK

Depo-Provera

Medroxyprogesterone acetate was licensed for short-term use until 1984. In 1984, a long-term licence for Depo-Provera was granted for use in women for whom other contraceptives are contraindicated or have caused unacceptable side-effects or are otherwise unsatisfactory. This method is now available in over 90 countries, including the USA.

Noristerat

Noristerat is presently licensed only for short-term use for women whose partners have undergone vasectomy until the vasectomy is effective, and for women immunised against rubella, to prevent pregnancy during the active period of the virus.

Advantages	▶ most effective method of family planning
	▶ one injection lasts for 8-12 weeks (depending on type)
	▶ non-intercourse related method
	▶ helpful for women with pre-menstrual symptoms and painful periods
	▶ safe, no deaths associated with this method.
	▶ minimal metabolic effects
	▶ no association with cardiovascular disease
	▶ can be used by breast-feeding mothers
	▶ most of the non-contraceptive benefits of combined oral contraceptives, including protection against PID

Disadvantages

▶ menstrual disturbances – bleeding may be frequent, irregular or absent

▶ weight gain (mainly associated with Depo-Provera)

▶ a long delay in the return of fertility (up to a year or more with Depo-Provera)

▶ depression in some women

▶ possible association with osteoporosis in some women (requires confirmation)

▶ cannot be withdrawn

Contra-indications

For *full* information see manufacturer's data sheet.

Injectable methods should not be given to women with:

▶ possible pregnancy

▶ cancer of the breast or undiagnosed breast lump

▶ all genital cancers (except as treatment for endometrial cancer)

▶ undiagnosed vaginal or uterine bleeding

▶ past severe arterial disease or current very high risk or severely abnormal lipid profile

▶ recent trophoblastic disease and elevated hCG levels

▶ serious side-effect on combined oral contraceptives, not clearly oestrogen attributable

▶ those women who cannot accept menstrual irregularity

▶ women who have had a baby and are breast-feeding should seek advice from their doctor as to when to start using this method

▶ women wishing to conceive immediately after use of injectable method

Periods

Most women using progestogen-only preparations experience some menstrual disturbance, which is not harmful. Injectables can cause irregular periods, spotting between periods or complete absence of periods (particularly after two or more injections). Menstrual irregularity is the main reason for discontinuation of this method. Women should be fully counselled about this when choosing injectable preparations.

Side-effects

The main reported side-effects include menstrual disturbances (see 'Periods' above), weight gain, headaches, some fluid retention, changes in mood, libido and depression in some women. Rare cases of thrombosis have been reported, but causality has not been established.

Planning a pregnancy

Many women experience a delay of return to fertility (more so with Depo-Provera) of up to a year or more. It should be noted that there is always a varying interval between women deciding to become pregnant and actual conception.

After childbirth and breast-feeding

Because of the risk of heavy or prolonged bleeding in some women, it is recommended that injectable methods in general *should not* be used until 5 to 6 weeks after childbirth due to increase in irregular bleeding. Injectable methods may safely be used while breast-feeding. Research on Depo-Provera has shown no deleterious effects on babies or infant growth or morbidity.

Drug interactions

There is little data on injectable methods and it is not known if injectable methods are affected by other medication in the same way as oral contraceptives. However, progestogens are known to be affected by enzyme inducing drugs (see 'Drugs and combined oral contraceptives' on page 44). Women taking enzyme inducing drugs should have their injection frequency increased from 12 to 10 weeks for Depo-Provera and from 8 to 6 weeks for Noristerat.

Monthly injectables and future methods

Research into improving injectable methods has been going on since the 1960s. Monthly injectables are available in some parts of the world. The World Health Organisation is currently researching a number of preparations, including progestogen-only injectable methods and combined oestrogen-progestogen methods.

Contraceptive implants

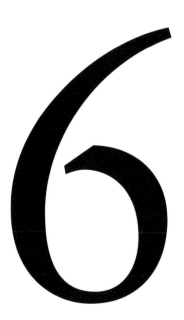

General information

Contraceptive implants offer an alternative way of delivering hormones that are long-acting, low-dose and reversible methods of contraception. A wide range of materials and approaches has beenused in the development of different hormonal delivery systems. Levonorgestrel is the most widely used hormone to date, but the newer progestogens may also prove valuable in the future.

The first contraceptive implant available in the UK is Norplant.This implant is widely used in other countries and the number of users worldwide exceeds two million women. Norplant is available in the same way as other contraceptive methods. Specialised training is *essential* for the success of this method.

Norplant consists of six thin flexible rods made of soft silastic. Each implant measures 34mm in length and 2.44mm in diameter. Each contains 38mg of levonorgestrel.

Using local anaesthesia, Norplant is inserted subdermally through a small incision using a trocar. The rods are positioned carefully in a fan shape in the inner aspect of the non-dominant arm, approximately 6-8cm above the fold of the elbow. Strict asepsis must be observed.

Once the implant is in place it is effective for 5 years. The implant can be removed at any time during this period. Providing the implants are correctly inserted, they will not move. Women should be reassured that they are not breakable.

Mode of action

Contraceptive implants work by preventing ovulation in about 50 per cent of menstrual cycles and by thickening the cervical mucus, preventing sperm penetration.

Efficacy

Contraceptive implants are highly effective. Norplant is almost 100 per cent effective in the first year of use, and about 98 per cent effective over 5 years.

Time of insertion	Implants should ideally be inserted on the first day of a menstrual cycle. No additional contraceptive methods are needed. If inserted on any other day, an additional contraceptive method is required for the first 7 days.

Advantages
- long-lasting
- very effective
- easily reversible and no effect on future fertility
- non-intercourse related
- free from oestrogen side-effects
- requires little medical attention other than at insertion and removal

Disadvantages
- requires an operative procedure
- irregular menstrual bleeding may occur
- possible risk of ectopic pregnancy (this will be a reduced risk compared to progestogen-only pills which have a higher overall failure rate)
- a small number of women will develop functional ovarian cysts

Contra-indications
- possible pregnancy
- active thromboembolic disorders
- undiagnosed uterine or liver disorder
- known or suspected cancer of the reproductive organs
- acute liver disease

Side-effects	Side-effects are similar to other progestogen-only methods. The possibility of irregular menstrual bleeding *must* be fully discussed.
Periods	Menstrual irregularity and disruption appear to be most common during the first year of use when the progestogen levels are highest. Irregular bleeding becomes less after the first year.
Planning a pregnancy	Implants can be removed at any point if a pregnancy is wanted. Fertility is not affected once the implant is removed.

Use after childbirth	Implants can be inserted from day 21 after childbirth. If inserted after this time, an additional contraceptive method should be used for 7 days. As implants are a new method, any long term effects relating to breast-feeding are not known. However, use of other progestogen-only methods are known to be safe.
Use after abortion or miscarriage	Implants can be used immediately after an early abortion or miscarriage.
Operations/ surgery	Progestogen implants need not be removed in the case of major surgery, but in cases of high risk thrombosis, consideration should be given to standard prophylactic measures.
Drug interactions	The guidelines for implants are the same as for combined and progestogen-only pills. Antibiotics do not reduce the effectiveness of progestogen-only methods.
Removal of implants	Norplant should be removed within 5 years of insertion. Removal can occur at any time in the menstrual cycle. Loss of contraceptive efficacy is immediate, so women should be appropriately advised. The implant is removed through a small incision using small forceps. If the method is to be continued, a new set of rods can be inserted through the incision but placed in the opposite direction.
Future types of implant	Several different types of hormonal implants are now being developed. Most involve fewer rods than Norplant, and will be effective for different lengths of time. Bio-degradable and non-biodegradable implants are being studied. Injectable microspheres and microcapsules are also being developed.

Intrauterine contraceptive devices

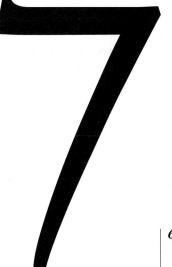

General information

Intrauterine contraceptive devices (IUDs) are small polyethylene and copper devices (some with silver cores) or polymer devices impregnated with medication (such as levonorgestrel-releasing IUDs). These come in varying shapes and sizes and are inserted into the uterus. Barium sulphate in the polyethylene makes the devices radio-opaque so they can be located, if necessary, by x-ray or ultrasound. Plastic IUDs (Lippes Loop and Saf-t-Coil) are no longer available now in the UK, but may still be in situ. All devices have monofilament threads for removal and to allow women to regularly check that the IUD is in position. They are effective for a number of years. See 'Duration of use' on page 70.

Mode of action

The antifertility effect of IUDs appears to be the result of a variety of mechanisms: the World Health Organisation (*Mechanism of action, safety and efficacy of intrauterine devices*, WHO, 1987) concluded:

'It is unlikely that the contraceptive efficacy of IUDs results, mainly or exclusively, from their capacity to interfere with implantation; it is more probable that they exert their antifertility effects beyond the uterus and interfere with steps in the reproductive process that take place before the ova reach the uterine cavity. It is likely that the uterine and tubal fluids that are altered in the presence of an IUD impair the viability of the gametes, thus reducing their chances of union and impeding fertilization. Copper ions released by an IUD probably potentiate these effects.'

All IUDs cause a foreign body reaction in the endometrium, with increased numbers of leucocytes. Hormone-releasing IUDs work in a similar way to other progestogen-only preparations, and may inhibit ovulation, in addition to the normal action of IUDs.

Table 6 gives a description of IUDs available in the UK.

Table 6 IUDs available in the UK

Type	Appearance	Manufacturer's recommended life span
Ortho Gyne-T Ortho (Cilag)	Copper wire on T-shaped polyethylene carrier with two monofilament threads Surface area of copper - 200 mm²	3 years*
Ortho Gyne-T 380S Ortho (Cilag)	Copper wire on T-shaped polyethylene carrier and copper on vertical section (320 mm²) and copper collars on each horizontal arm (30 mm²) Two monofilament threads	4 years*
Novagard Kabi **Nova-T** Schering	Copper wire with silver core on T-shaped polyethylene carrier with two monofilament threads Surface area of copper - 200 mm²	5 years*
Multiload Cu250 Organon	Copper wire on polyethylene carrier with flexible U-shaped side arms with two monofilament threads Surface area of copper - 250 mm²	3 years*
Multiload Cu250 Short Organon	Copper wire on polyethylene carrier with flexible U-shaped side arms with two monofilament threads Surface area of copper - 250 mm²	3 years*
Multiload Cu375 Organon	Copper wire on polyethylene carrier with flexible U-shaped side arms with two monofilament threads Surface area of copper - 375 mm²	5 years*

* See 'Duration of use' on page 70

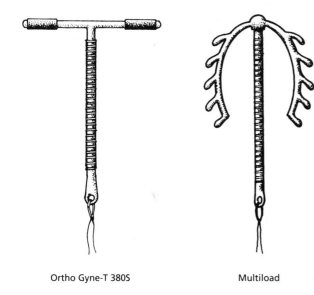

Ortho Gyne-T 380S   Multiload

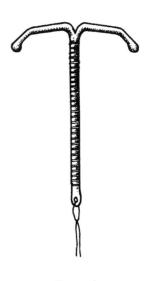

Novagard
Nova-T

Efficacy

IUDs are highly effective methods and benefit from no 'user' failures. Today's modern IUDs have very low failure rates compared to the earlier first generation (plastic only) IUDs. The general effectiveness of IUDs ranges from between 98 to almost 100 per cent. The newer third generation devices with larger surface areas of copper such as the Ortho Gyne-T 380S have failure rates of less than 1 per 100 after one year of use. After the first year of use, most devices have a lower failure rate.

Advantages

▶ provides long term, highly effective, reversible contraception
▶ effective immediately after fitting
▶ non-intercourse related
▶ requires no daily action or remembering
▶ ideal for women over 25 who are spacing their pregnancies
▶ very low mortality/morbidity

Disadvantages

▶ may cause menstrual irregularities with inter-menstrual bleeding and spotting
▶ periods may be heavier at first and more painful
▶ sometimes the IUD may be expelled
▶ some women develop a pelvic infection, risk appears to be highest in the first few months after insertion. Pelvic infection is more likely in younger and nulliparous women, and in women who are not in stable monogamous relationships, who are at risk of STDs
▶ there are other extremely rare complications, eg perforation
▶ not ideal for young women (under 25) who have not had children
▶ there is a risk of ectopic pregnancy in the event of IUD failure (there is less risk with IUDs releasing copper with a surface area of more than 300mm²; any risk is still less than in women not using contraception)

Contra-indications

For *full* information see manufacturer's data sheets.

▶ known or suspected pregnancy
▶ any undiagnosed abnormal uterine or vaginal bleeding

- menorrhagia (heavy bleeding)
- present pelvic inflammatory disease (or possible past infection)
- heart valve replacement
- distorted uterine cavity
- immunosuppressive therapy
- previous ectopic pregnancy, or high risk for ectopic pregnancy (eg tubal surgery)
- copper allergy (this is rare)
- women who are not in stable monogamous relationships

Administration

IUDs should only be fitted by doctors trained in fitting and inserting IUDs. The selection of clients, the timing and skill of insertion and the choice of device is critical to the success of IUDs and can affect how an IUD is accepted, as well as determine its continuation of use.

Good resuscitation facilities should be available *and* known about.

Timing of insertion

IUDs may be inserted up to day 19 of a 28 day menstrual cycle. The usual time is at the end of a period, when the bleeding is less and the cervix is softer and more dilated. Also it is obvious that a woman is not pregnant.

Using the IUD after childbirth

In the UK, IUDs are not normally fitted immediately after childbirth as there tends to be a higher risk of expulsion. Postpartum IUD insertion usually occurs at about six weeks after birth. However, immediate post-delivery insertion can be carried out (if there is no puerperal infection or any other contraindications) in skilled hands providing a woman is not breast-feeding. Breast-feeding may increase the risk of perforation. After Caesarian delivery, the normal practice is to defer insertion to at least six to eight weeks after birth.

Using the IUD after abortion or miscarriage

An IUD can be inserted immediately after an early (first trimester) abortion or miscarriage. If it is not inserted immediately, it should be fitted 4 to 6 weeks later.

Using the IUD after unprotected intercourse

The IUD can be used as a postcoital contraceptive within five days of unprotected intercourse (see 'Emergency contraception' on page 115).

Instructions for use

Once the IUD is fitted, a woman should be taught to feel the IUD threads which come through the cervix. This enables a woman to check that her IUD is in place. This should be done regularly each month after the end of a period. If the strings cannot be felt, or if the plastic end of the IUD can be felt, this should be checked immediately, as this might mean the IUD is being expelled.

Any continued bleeding, pain or unusual vaginal discharge should be checked out by vaginal examination.

Duration of use

Modern copper IUDs have varying life spans of three to five years, depending on the type of IUD. These differ from country to country and tend to be the minimum lifespans. Extensive clinical research shows that for many devices the lifespan exceeds the manufacturer's recommendations. The Medical Advisory Committees of the Family Planning Association (FPA) and the Faculty of Family Planning and Reproductive Health Care recommend that for routine management modern third generation copper-bearing

An IUD in place

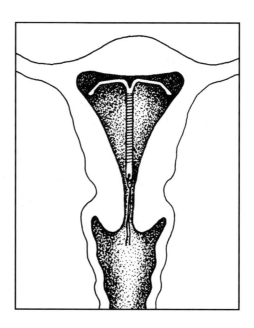

IUDs may be left in place for a *minimum* of 5 years. IUDs inserted after the age of 40 can be left in until the menopause. Plastic IUDs still in situ can be left in until the menopause in the absence of any problems.

Side-effects

Bleeding problems

The occurrence of irregular bleeding or heavier and longer periods, particularly in the first couple of months can be one of the main problems of IUDs for some women. Bleeding and some discomfort in the first couple of days after insertion is quite normal. Any pain (similar to period pains) can be controlled by simple analgesics. Any unusual bleeding, pain or discharge should always be investigated.

Pelvic infection

Pelvic inflammatory disease (PID) is the general term for infection of the upper genital tract, including the uterus, fallopian tubes and ovaries. There is extensive research on the association between use of IUDs and PID. Much of it is inconclusive. However, it is generally considered that the overall risk of PID in IUD users is in the range of 1.5 to 2.6. Risks appear to be highest in the first few months after IUD insertion. The main factors that increase the risk of getting PID are parity, age and sexual activity. Because of the association of PID with multiple partners, it is not a recommended method for women who are not in a *mutually* faithful sexual relationship.

Modern copper IUDs are associated with lower risks of PID than the older inert devices.

Infection may be associated with pain during or after intercourse, unusual vaginal discharge, lower abdominal or back pain or irregular bleeding. Immediate treatment is necessary to minimise any damage to the reproductive tract.

Actinomyces-like organisms (ALOs) in cervical smears

The medical advice and clinical management today is that where this occurs in an asymptomatic woman:

▶ the device should normally be removed, using careful technique to avoid vaginal contamination of the main part of the device
▶ the tails of the removed device should be cut off with sterile scissors and discarded. The main body of the device is then dropped into a sterile container and sent for culture for actinomyces. The device should not be refrigerated but should be sent to the laboratory as quickly as possible. It is useful to use a laboratory, such as that in a dental hospital, which is accustomed to performing actinomyces cultures.
▶ a fresh device can be inserted immediately
▶ the cervical smear should be repeated in three months
▶ in the rare event of actinomyces being cultured from the body of the device, the woman should be treated with Amoxicillin 3 grams daily for 90 days, even if asymptomatic. If she has an IUD, it should be removed, as it is contraindicated in the presence, or past history, of actinomycosis infection. She should not use an IUD as a method in the future.
▶ if the culture is negative, as is most likely, no treatment is required, but follow up with cervical smears is recommended
▶ if it is impossible to have the removed device cultured, immediate refitting is advised with careful follow up and cervical smears at 3 months

Perforation

Perforation where the IUD penetrates through the cervix or the uterus is uncommon (the risk is about one in a thousand insertions). This may happen at insertion, or be diagnosed later. Any pain or discomfort either after insertion or later should always be checked immediately to rule out perforation or any other problem.

Expulsion

This problem relates to all IUD types. The risk is greatest in the first 3 months after insertion. Expulsion is more common in nulliparous women. Women should be encouraged to check the IUD strings carefully in the first few months, and then once a month, after the end of each period.

Missing or lost threads

If the threads cannot be felt during a monthly check the woman should be advised to return to her doctor, and advised not to rely on her IUD until this has been checked. An additional contraceptive method should be used during this time. Missing threads may indicate pregnancy, or that the device has been expelled, or that the threads have been withdrawn up into the uterus, or that the IUD has moved. There are various ways this can be checked, all requiring a skilled practitioner or specialist centre.

Pregnancy with an IUD in place

Any suspected pregnancy should be investigated immediately. A pregnancy may be extrauterine or intrauterine. Extrauterine pregnancy (ectopic pregnancy) is a serious problem, and requires immediate referral. An ectopic pregnancy may be associated with a light, scanty or missed period, usually with lower abdominal pain.

Intrauterine pregnancy with an IUD in place may go successfully to term or miscarry. Where possible, if the choice is to continue with the pregnancy the IUD should be removed. Removal of the IUD should be attempted only if the pregnancy is less than 12 weeks advanced, and the threads are easily visible and offer no resistance to removal. (In the absence of visible threads, ultrasound can be used.) The risk of miscarriage is higher (over 50 per cent) if the IUD is left in place, than if it is removed (where the miscarriage rate is about 20 per cent). There is no evidence of any abnormality in the baby, if the pregnancy goes to term. (If the IUD is removed the miscarriage rate is about 20 per cent). The IUD is usually expelled with the afterbirth as it is positioned outside the gestational sac containing the baby. If it is not expelled with the afterbirth, location of the device is essential. It should not be assumed that it was expelled at an earlier time.

Drug interactions

Antibiotic therapy does not interfere with copper IUDs.

Reports that the use of anti-inflammatory drugs such as aspirin and corticosteroids increases the failure rate of IUDs has not been confirmed, but corticosteroid therapy may increase the suseptibility to infection.

Diathermy

Short wave diathermy is not a contraindication in IUD users, but is considered a theoretical risk and so caution is advised.

Follow-up

Regular check-ups are advised. After insertion of the IUD a woman should be seen within the first 2 weeks or sooner if there is a problem, then after 6 months, and then yearly. If a woman wishes to become pregnant, the IUD is easily removed and there is no detrimental effect on fertility.

New IUDs

Hormonal releasing IUDs such as Levonova should be available within the next couple of years. This levo-norgestrel-releasing T-shaped IUD is associated with extremely few side effects including protection against ectopic pregnancy. It has very low pregnancy rates – less that 0.5 per 100 women per year. It lasts for a minimum of 5 years. In addition to its contraceptive effects, its use in other therapeutic areas such as menorrhagia and hormone replacement make the levonorgestrel-releasing IUD an important new method for the future.

Other IUDs being researched include modified designs, such as flexible and frameless IUDs, to help reduce expulsion and other side-effects associated with current IUDs.

Female barrier methods –
Diaphragm, cap, female condom

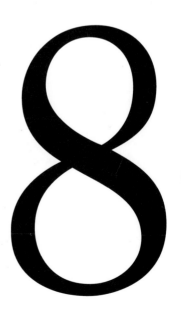

General information

There is now a variety of female barrier methods to choose from. These include, diaphragms, caps and female condoms. Diaphragms and caps should always be used with *spermicides.*

Diaphragms and caps

Diaphragms and caps are available from family planning clinics, family doctors and pharmacies.

Mode of action

They fit into the vagina and cover the cervix to provide a barrier between the egg and sperm, so preventing fertilisation.

Efficacy

When used carefully and correctly with spermicide, diaphragms and caps have an effectiveness rate of 85-98 per cent.

Products available

See Table 7.

Diaphragms

Diaphragms, commonly known as caps are thin soft latex rubber, dome-shaped devices with a flexible circular ring covered by rubber. They come in different sizes from 55mm to 100mm rising in 5mm steps. They fit into the vagina between the posterior fornix and behind the pubic bone to cover the cervix. The diaphragm is held in place by the vaginal muscles, the tension of the ring and the pubic bone. There are three types of diaphragm.

Flat spring
The rim contains a firm, flat watch-spring metal band and squeezes flat for insertion. These diaphragms are suitable for women with normal vaginas, and are usually offered first. They come in sizes of 55-95mm.

Coil spring
The rim contains a round spiral of coiled metal wire. It is more flexible than the flat spring type. Where a flat spring diaphragm is not suitable, a coil spring should be

tried, providing the woman has good vaginal muscle tone. Because they are more flexible they can be more comfortable than the flat spring. They come in sizes of 55-100mm.

Arcing spring
These combine the features of the coil and flat spring diaphragm. It squeezes into an arc for insertion. They provide a useful alternative for women who have poor vaginal muscular support, or where the length or the position of the cervix makes fitting of a coil spring or flat spring diaphragm more difficult. They come in sizes of 60-95mm.

Caps

Caps are smaller than diaphragms. They are made of rubber and fit directly over the cervix. They are held in place mainly by suction and by support from the vaginal wall. They come in different shapes and sizes. Caps are a useful alternative for women who wish to use a barrier method, but cannot use diaphragms. They deserve to be better promoted by professionals.

Cervical cap (Prentif cavity rim)
This is a thick rim cervical cap. It is a deep soft cap which is shaped like a thimble with a firm rim and groove around the inner lip of the rim. This provides the suction. It comes in four sizes ranging from 22mm to 31mm, rising in 3mm steps.

Vault cap (Dumas cap)
This is a semi-circular shallow dome-shaped cap, which comes in five sizes ranging from 55mm to 75mm, rising in 5mm steps.

Vimule cap
This combines the features of the cervical and vault cap. It is dome-shaped with a thinner splayed rim which adheres to the vaginal walls. It comes in three sizes ranging from 45mm to 51mm.

Table 7 Diaphragms and caps

Product & manufacturer	Description	Colour	Size
Diaphragms			
Durex LRC	Flat spring diaphragm	Opaque	55-95mm (rising in 5mm steps)
Ortho Ortho (Cilag)	Coil spring diaphragm	Opaque	55-100mm (rising in 5mm steps)
Ortho Ortho (Cilag)	Flat spring diaphragm	White	55-95mm (rising in 5mm steps)
All Flex Ortho (Cilag)	Arcing spring diaphragm	Opaque	60-95mm (rising in 5mm steps)
Durex Arcing Spring LRC	Arcing spring diaphragm	Opaque	60-95mm (rising in 5mm steps)
Caps			
Dumas Lamberts (Dalston)	Vault cap	Translucent or caramel/cream	55-75mm (rising in 5mm steps)
Prentif Cavity Rim Lamberts (Dalston)	Cervical cap	Caramel/cream	22-31mm (rising in 3mm steps)
Vimule Cap Lamberts (Dalston)	Vimule cap	Translucent	45-51mm (3 sizes)

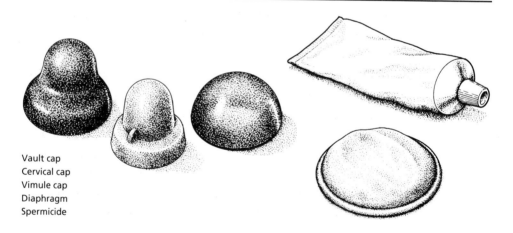

Vault cap
Cervical cap
Vimule cap
Diaphragm
Spermicide

Advantages

▶ very effective with careful use
▶ can be put in at any convenient time before having sex so it need not interfere with spontaneity
▶ may protect against cancer of the cervix, some sexually transmitted diseases (STDs, although not HIV) and pelvic inflammatory disease
▶ there are no established health risks or side-effects
▶ under the direct control of the woman

Disadvantages
- requires thinking ahead so that the diaphragm/cap is in place or readily available
- requires careful use for it to be effective
- an increased incidence of cystitis or urinary tract infection in some women using diaphragms
- must be used with spermicides

Contra-indications
- very poor muscle tone may be a contraindication for the diaphragm
- women with a shallow pubic ledge – this applies to the diaphragm only
- abnormality of the vagina
- women who are unable to touch their genital area with comfort
- any irritation, sensitivity or allergy to latex or spermicides
- a present vaginal, cervical or pelvic infection, or recurrent urinary tract infection
- past toxic shock syndrome
- lack of privacy for insertion, removal or care of the diaphragm/cap

Administration

Diaphragms and caps are free on prescription on the NHS. In addition, they can be obtained without prescription by buying them from pharmacies (the size will need to be known). They should be fitted and their use taught by a trained family planning nurse or doctor. The acceptability of diaphragms and caps is much higher if women are taught by enthusiastic, trained personnel. They should always be used with spermicides, see 'Spermicides' on page 93.

Instructions for use of diaphragms and caps

The correct size and type for an individual women can only be determined by vaginal examination. Full instructions should be given on how to use and care for the diaphragm or cap.

The diaphragm or cap with spermicide can be inserted at *any time* before having sex. If it is inserted more than 3 hours before intercourse, or if intercourse occurs more

Inserting a diaphragm

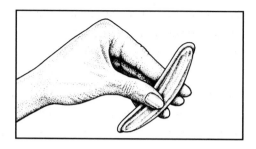

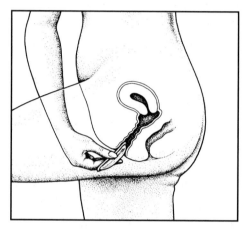

Diaphragm in position

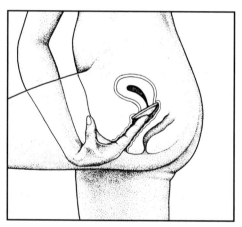

Cap in position

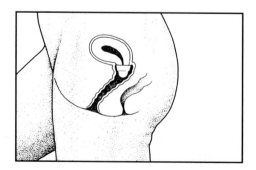

than once, additional spermicide should be used without removing the diaphragm or cap. They must be used at all times with a spermicide. The diaphragm or cap must be left in place for at least 6 hours after intercourse, but should not be left in the vagina for longer than 30 hours (this will include the 6 hours after use). Providing the diaphragm or cap is correctly inserted, neither partner should be able to feel it. If it can be felt or is uncomfortable a woman should have it checked by her doctor or clinic. For some women, the use of an introducer can help with the insertion of a diaphragm.

All oil-based products, such as petroleum jelly, baby oils, bath oils etc, should be avoided with latex products as they cause rapid deterioration of rubber. Oil-based vaginal and rectal medications should also be avoided. After use, the diaphragm or cap should be washed with mild unscented soap, well rinsed and dried carefully. It should be stored in a cool place. It should be checked for any holes or deterioration before each use.

Practice diaphragms or caps are usually given to women when they first choose to use these methods. Women must be advised that practice diaphragms or caps should not be relied on as contraceptives. Their purpose is to allow a woman to feel confident about using the method before actively relying on it as a method of birth control.

Using diaphragms or caps after childbirth The diaphragm or cap can be used about 6 weeks after childbirth, after vaginal muscle tone is restored. A woman should always be checked for size after childbirth.

Using diaphragms or caps after an abortion or miscarriage The diaphragm or cap should be checked for size after an abortion or miscarriage as the vagina may change in shape or size.

Duration of use Diaphragms or caps should be replaced annually, or immediately if any problem such as holes or puckering of the rubber occurs. Discoloration will occur, and is quite normal; it does not affect the latex.

83

Side-effects

There are few side-effects with these methods.

Irritation

Some women do have increased sensitivity, irritation or allergy to latex or spermicides. It is important that any symptoms are always checked out to rule out any pre-existing or new vaginal infection.

Urinary tract infection

There is some indication that some women who use diaphragms develop cystitis and urethritis more frequently than women who use other methods. This may be due to pressure on the urethra, especially if the diaphragm is too big. If this is a recurrent problem, the size of the diaphragm should be carefully checked and if necessary, one of the smaller caps should be tried.

Toxic shock syndrome

A few cases of toxic shock syndrome have been reported in diaphragm users. Almost all cases have been in women who have worn the diaphragm for *more than 30 hours.*

Follow-up

Diaphragms and caps should be replaced annually, and checked for size and fitting. They should also be automatically checked after childbirth, abortion or miscarriage or if a woman gains or loses 3kg (7lb) in weight.

Future types of barrier method

Research is being carried out into producing different kinds of cervical barriers, which may offer methods that are more effective, easier to fit and can be used without spermicides.

Female condoms

General information

The female condom is a lubricated, loose fitting polyurethane sheath with two flexible rings, which is inserted into the vagina. It lines the vagina and covers some of the vulva. It comes in one size and does not need to be fitted by a health professional. Female condoms are available from family planning clinics, pharmacies, by mail order and from other retail outlets.

Mode of action The female condom acts as a barrier between sperm and egg, so preventing fertilisation.

Efficacy At present there are no large studies showing ranges of the effectiveness rates. Most opinion suggests it will be as effective as the male condom which has an effectiveness rate of 85-98 per cent.

Products available At present there is only one female condom available in the UK. It is called Femidom. A number of similar products are being researched.

Advantages ▶ no known side effects
▶ it acts as both a contraceptive and prophylactic against STDs, including HIV, and may protect against cancer of the cervix and PID
▶ effective with careful use
▶ under the direct control of the woman
▶ can be used at any time before having sex
▶ does not require additional spermicide
▶ can be used with oil-based products

Disadvantages ▶ requires thought before use
▶ not so discreetly disposable as male condoms
▶ requires careful insertion and use for it to be effective
▶ can interrupt sex

Contra-indications ▶ women who are unable to touch their genital area with comfort
▶ women with a pre-existing vaginal or cervical infection

Instructions for use If obtained from a family planning clinic, a nurse or doctor can provide instructions on how to use the female condom. If bought at a pharmacy, full instructions are available with the packet. Each female condom is individually packaged. The condom is inserted into the vagina using the inner ring as a guide. The condom should be pushed up behind the pubic bone. The inner ring, as well as acting as a guide, keeps it in place. The outer ring lies flat against the body covering the vulva and helps prevent the condom from being drawn down into the vagina during intercourse. When correctly in place, the condom should loosely line the vagina and feel comfortable. It can be inserted any time before having sex. Like all barrier methods, there should be no genital contact before or after use. Care needs to be taken that the penis is not inserted between the outside of the condom and the vaginal wall. The condom should be used only once. Additional spermicides or lubricants of any type can be used (unlike with latex products). If the method is not used correctly, then advice regarding emergency contraception should be obtained.

Male barrier methods – Male condom

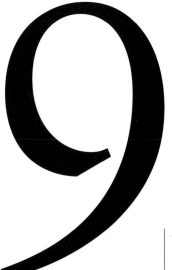

General information

The male condom is one of the oldest methods of family planning, and apart from vasectomy (male sterilisation), it is the only reliable method a man can use. Male condoms are currently made of natural latex. Condoms are available free from family planning clinics. They are not generally available from family doctors. They are available to buy from a variety of sources: pharmacies, retail outlets, by mail order and from garages and vending machines.

Mode of action

The male condom, which fits over the erect penis, acts as a barrier between egg and sperm, so preventing fertilisation.

Efficacy

Male condoms, when used carefully and consistently, are highly effective in preventing both pregnancy and sexually transmitted infections, including HIV. Their general effectiveness ranges from about 85-98 per cent.

Main products available

See Table 8.

The FPA recommends only condoms which are certified to British Standards Institution (BSI) specification (BS 3704). Products that have passed these standards are recognised by the Kitemark. The BSI Kitemark scheme of product quality certification requires manufacturers to satisfy the BSI that the entire manufacturing system from raw materials to goods leaving the premises complies with the recognised standard of good manufacturing practice. The use of the Kitemark illustrates a reliable quality product. Many condom products are imported into the UK and sold with claims of 'made to BS 3704' or 'tested to BS 3704', these *do not* have BSI approval and *should not* be recommended.

After many years of work, a European and an International standard is now available for male condoms.

Table 8 lists only the main BSI Kitemarked condoms.

Table 8 Main varieties of Kitemarked condoms available in the UK

Product & manufacturer	Presentation	Description
LRC Products (Durex)		
Spermicidally lubricated		
Safe-Play	Lightweight, transparent, teat-ended	Packets of 3, 10
Safe-Play Ribbed	Teat-ended, transparent, ribbed	Packets of 3, 10
Extra Safe	Coral, teat-ended, anatomically shaped	Packets of 3, 12, 18
Elite	Transparent, teat-ended	Packets of 3, 12, 18
Fetherlight	Transparent, teat-ended, thinnest Durex condom	Packets of 3, 12, 18
Arouser	Coral, teat-ended, ribbed	Packets of 3, 12
Gold	Gold, plain-ended	Packets of 3, 12
Assure	Coral, teat-ended	Packets of 3 x 2
Lubricated (non-spermicidal)		
Gossamer	Transparent, teat-ended	Packets of 3, 12, 18
Safe-Play Coloured	Red and blue, teat-ended	Packet of 2
Safe-Play Black	Black, teat-ended	Packet of 2
Extra Strong	Thickest Durex condom, transparent, plain-ended	Packets of 6
Allergy	Transparent, teat-ended, hypoallergenic	Packets of 3, 12
Unlubricated		
Safe-Play Minty	Green, mint-flavoured, teat-ended	Packet of 2
Mates Healthcare*		
Spermicidally lubricated		
Mates Contoured	Transparent, contoured, teat-ended	Packets of 3, 12
Mates Natural	Transparent, flared, teat-ended	Packets of 3, 12
Mates Superstrong	Transparent, straight, teat-ended	Packets of 3, 12
Mates Play	Coloured, straight, ribbed, teat-ended	Packets of 3, 12
Mates Coloured	Coloured, contoured, teat-ended	Packets of 3
Lady Mates	Transparent, contoured, teat-ended	Packets of 3
Lubricated (non-spermicidal)		
Mates Natural	Transparent, flared, teat-ended	Packets of 3
Mates Superstrong	Transparent, straight, teat-ended	Packets of 3
Mates Snugger Fitting	Transparent, contoured, teat-ended	Packets of 3
Unlubricated		
Mates Mint Fragrance	Transparent, flared, mint-flavoured, teat-ended	Packets of 3, 12

* Johnson & Johnson is the retail distributor of Mates, and Sutherland Health Ltd is the NHS distributor. **Note**: other varieties of BSI Kitemarked condoms, such as Jiffi brands distributed by Sime Health UK Ltd, are available in the UK.

Condoms come in a variety of types: unlubricated, lubricated with silicone or spermicide, coloured, ribbed, teat-ended, plain-ended, shaped, non-flavoured or flavoured. Spermicidally lubricated condoms in the UK contain Nonoxynol 9.

Advantages

▶ no side-effects
▶ very effective with careful use
▶ easy to obtain and use
▶ the man can take the responsibility for birth control
▶ can protect either partner against some sexually transmitted diseases, including HIV
▶ may protect the woman against cancer of the cervix and PID
▶ requires no medical supervision

Disadvantages

▶ requires forward planning each time
▶ needs to be used carefully to be effective
▶ possible loss of sensitivity during intercourse
▶ may interrupt sex, although putting on the condom can be enjoyed as part of foreplay
▶ needs to be disposed of carefully
▶ cannot be used with oil-base products

Contra-indications

▶ any allergy, irritation or sensitivity to latex or spermicide
▶ men unable to maintain erection during intercourse

Instructions for use

If male condoms are provided through a family planning clinic, family planning nurses or doctors can advise on correct usage of the condom. Full instructions also come with packets if obtained elsewhere.

Like all barrier methods, condoms must be used before any genital contact. To use the condom, the closed or teat end of the condom is squeezed to expel any air and leaves about a centimetre to receive the ejaculated semen. It is then rolled down over the full length of the erect penis. After ejaculation the condom should be carefully removed holding it firmly at the rim as the penis is withdrawn.

Male condoms should be used only once. The expiry date on the packet should be checked and all oil based products should be avoided with latex products. Certain vaginal and rectal medications should also be avoided.

Additional spermicide products of any type can be used if required.

Skin condoms are available to buy, but they are not BSI Kitemarked and are not recommended by the FPA as either contraceptives or prophylactics. Currently, there are no plastic-only condoms.

It is generally assumed that everyone knows how to use condoms, but this is not the case. Health professionals are in an ideal position to help with any concerns or queries.

Side-effects

There are no adverse side-effects of male condoms except possible sensitivity, irritation or allergy to the latex or spermicide. If this is a problem a non-spermicidally lubricated or hypoallergenic type is recommended.

Future types of condoms

Research is currently being carried out into different varieties of condoms, including some made of different kinds of polymers, to improve sensitivity and user acceptability.

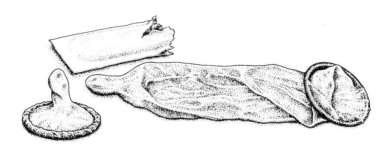

Spermicides

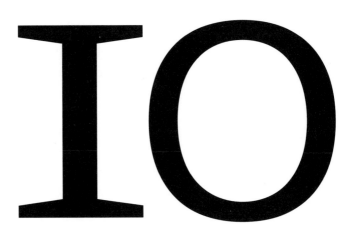

General information

Spermicides are chemical compounds in the form of aerosol foams, jellies, creams, films or pessaries that are inserted into the vagina prior to intercourse. They are not effective as a sole contraceptive method and are generally used with barrier methods. The vaginal contraceptive sponge is a carrier of spermicide (see 'The vaginal contraceptive sponge' on page 97).

Mode of action

The main chemical constituent in UK spermicide preparations is Nonoxynol 9 in an inert base. Spermicides kill sperm mainly by altering the integrity of the sperm cell membrane. In addition, the vaginal pH is altered providing an inhospitable environment for sperm.

Products available

See Table 9.

Advantages

▶ no serious side effects
▶ easily available and simple to use
▶ provides lubrication
▶ provides some protection against STDs, including HIV
▶ enhances efficacy of barrier methods

Disadvantages

▶ should not be used as sole contraceptive
▶ possible sensitivity, irritation or allergy
▶ can be perceived as messy

Instructions for use

All spermicide products should be used in conjunction with barrier methods. Use and efficacy of spermicides vary according to the type used. Type of spermicide, perfume and lubricating properties may influence choice. Applicators for some creams, jellies and foams are available.

Side-effects

There are few side-effects due to spermicides. Allergy is rare; sensitivity or irritation is more common. If sensitivity or irritation occur, another brand (with a different pH) should be tried. Any existing vaginal infection should be checked out as this can be exacerbated by spermicide use. Research shows no adverse effects on the fetus if spermicides are inadvertently used during pregnancy.

Table 9 Spermicide products

Products & manufacturer/ distributor	Chemical constituents	pH	Presentation	
Foams supplied in aerosol containers, with or without an applicator				
Delfen Foam Ortho (Cilag)	Nonoxynol 9, 12.5% in a water miscible base	4.5-5.0	20g with applicator refill 20g	
Creams supplied in metal tubes				
Ortho-Creme Ortho (Cilag)	Nonoxynol 9, 2% in a water miscible base	6.0	70g	*
Duracreme LRC	Nonoxynol 9, 2%	6.0-7.0	100g	*
Jellies supplied in metal tubes				
Duragel LRC	Nonoxynol 9, 2%	6.0-7.0	100g	*
Ortho-Gynol Jelly Ortho (Cilag)	Di-isobutylphenoxy- polyethoxyethanol, 1% in a water soluble base	4.5	81g	*
Gynol II Ortho (Cilag)	Nonoxynol 9, 2% in a water soluble base	4.5-4.7	81g	*
Staycept Jelly Syntex	Octoxynol (polyoxyethylene-octylphenol), 1%	4.25-4.75	80g	
Pessaries				
Ortho-Forms Ortho (Cilag)	Nonoxynol 9, 5% in a water soluble base	4.0-5.0	15 individually sealed pessaries	
Staycept pessaries Syntex	Nonoxynol 9, 6% in a water soluble base	4.25-5.25	10 individually sealed pessaries	
Double Check FP Sales	Nonoxynol 9, 6% in a water soluble base	4.25-5.25	10 individually sealed pessaries	
Films				
C Film FP Sales	Nonoxynol 9, 67mg in water soluble film	5.0-7.0	Packets of 10 5cm square films	

* Separate applicator available

Future methods Research is being carried out into the development of more effective, longer-acting spermicides with different base materials.

The vaginal contraceptive sponge

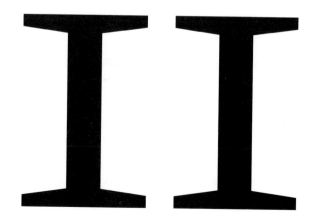

General information

The contraceptive sponge is a soft, circular sponge made of polyurethane foam. It is impregnated with Nonoxynol 9. It comes in a single size and measures about 5.5cm in diameter and 2.5cm thick, and has a fixed ribbon to facilitate removal. It is available from some family planning clinics and from pharmacies as an over-the-counter product.

Mode of action

The sponge acts as a carrier of spermicide, which is activated when moistened. In addition to its spermicidal action, it absorbs semen and, to a lesser extent, covers the cervix. It is not considered to be a barrier method.

Efficacy

The effectiveness of the sponge ranges from 75 to 91 per cent. It is not generally recommended because of its high failure rate. However, it may be chosen by women nearing the menopause and by women who are breast-feeding, when fertility is reduced.

Products available

The only product available in the UK is marketed under the name 'Today'.

Advantages

▶ one size is suitable for all women
▶ no fitting is required (though teaching of the method is desirable)
▶ non-intercourse related
▶ no mess attached to its use
▶ easily available from pharmacies
▶ it can be worn for 24 hours, allowing repeated intercourse
▶ few side effects

Disadvantages

▶ high failure rate
▶ possible irritation, sensitivity or allergy to the spermicide
▶ not as discreetly disposable as male condoms
▶ expensive

Contra-indications

▶ women who must not get pregnant
▶ possible sensitivity, irritation or allergy to spermicides
▶ existing vaginal infection
▶ women who cannot touch their genital area with comfort

Instructions for use

If obtained from a family planning clinic, instruction for use can be obtained from the family planning nurse or doctor. Full instructions come with the packet if obtained elsewhere. Moistened with water to activate the spermicide, the sponge is placed high in the vagina over the cervix. It can be used for more than one act of intercourse, and must be left in place for 6 hours after the last intercourse. It should not be left in place for more than 30 hours (this will include the 6 hours after intercourse). It should be not be used during a period. The sponge has an attached ribbon to facilitate removal. It should be disposed of carefully, not thrown down the toilet.

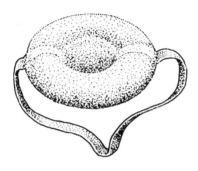

Natural family planning or fertility awareness methods

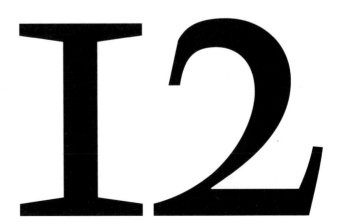

General information

The traditional terms 'rhythm' and 'safe period' to designate family planning based on the detection of ovulation have been replaced over the last decade by the terms 'natural family planning' (NFP) or 'fertility awareness' methods. These methods are based on the recognition of the naturally occurring signs and symptoms of ovulation identifying the fertile and infertile phases of the menstrual cycle in order to plan or prevent a pregnancy. Learning about fertility awareness provides a woman with good understanding of her body.

Natural family planning methods

There are four main methods:

▶ the temperature method
▶ the cervical mucus method
▶ the calendar method
▶ combination of methods: sympto-thermal method or double-check method

How natural family planning methods work

All these methods are intended to help to recognise or predict the timing of ovulation, by identifying the fertile and infertile phases of the menstrual cycle. Ovulation is the result of a complex and delicate sequence of events in the body, which occur 12-16 days *before* a woman's next period. The egg remains capable of being fertilised for about 12-24 hours and some sperm may be capable of fertilising an egg for about 3-5 days. Thus, the fertile phase is a relatively short time each month.

The temperature method

This relies on the measurement of normal changes in body temperature that occur after ovulation. Immediately after ovulation, basal body temperature (BBT – the body's temperature at complete rest) drops slightly and then rises by about 0.2°C to 0.4°C. It stays high until just before the next period.

The cervical mucus method

This relies on the detection of changes in cervical mucus which occur during the menstrual cycle. By noting the changes between 'infertile' and 'fertile' mucus, ovulation can be predicted and detected.

The calendar method

This involves working out the probability of the fertile time in advance each month based on the calculations of six to twelve menstrual cycles. This is no longer recognised as a reliable single indicator of fertility, as it makes no allowance for cycle irregularity, stress, illness, etc.

The sympto-thermal method

This combines all the indicators of fertility. This is often referred to as the double-check method. Some women know intuitively whether they are fertile from a number of physical and emotional changes occurring in the two weeks before a period is due. For example, changes occurring in the position and softness of the cervix, mid-cycle pain (mittelschmerz), discharge or bleeding, breast sensitivity or mood changes. Women may experience some or all of these changes.

Efficacy

The sympto-thermal method is the most effective of the NFP methods. The effectiveness ranges from 80 to 98 per cent.

Advantages

▶ can be used to plan a pregnancy as well as prevent conception
▶ there are no known physical side-effects
▶ non-intercourse related method
▶ couples share responsibility for family planning and may become more aware of how their bodies work
▶ some couples feel they enjoy intercourse more after abstaining during the fertile time
▶ no mechanical devices or hormones are used
▶ it may be the only acceptable method for some couples whose religious or personal beliefs prevent them from using other methods of family planning
▶ once the method has been learned by the user, no further follow-up or expense is necessary

Disadvantages
- it requires the commitment of both partners
- the methods require careful observation and record keeping, which may take time to learn
- for successful use of these methods, teaching is required from specially trained NFP teachers
- high motivation is required

Sources of help

Unfortunately good NFP teaching is seldom available from community family planning clinics or in general practice. Specialist help, including a list of trained NFP teachers, can be obtained from The Natural Family Planning Service and The National Association of Natural Family Planning Teachers (see 'Addresses of useful organisations' on page 154 for more details).

Summary illustration of fertility awareness methods

Days of cycle

1	2	3	4	5	6	7	8	9	10	11	12	13	14	15	16	17	18	19	20	21	22	23	24	25	26	27	28	1	2

Calendar method

safe period	unsafe period (for a woman whose cycle varies from 25-31 days)	safe period

Mucus method

bleeding	dry	mucus increases and gets clearer	mucus decreases and gets cloudy	dry

at ovulation mucus resembles
the white of a raw egg

Temperature method

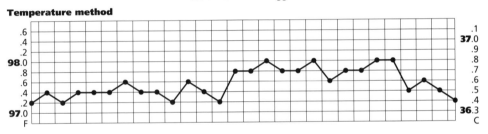

Ovary

growth of follicle   ovulation   corpus luteum

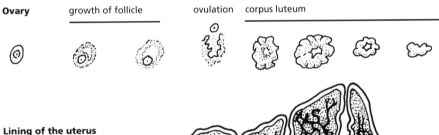

Lining of the uterus

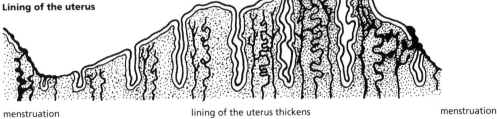

menstruation   lining of the uterus thickens   menstruation

1	2	3	4	5	6	7	8	9	10	11	12	13	14	15	16	17	18	19	20	21	22	23	24	25	26	27	28	1	2

Sterilisation

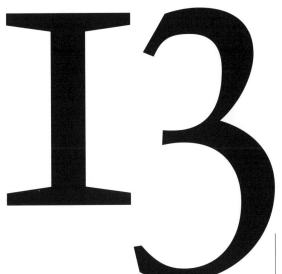

Sterilisation involves cutting, sealing or blocking the fallopian tubes in the woman, or the vas deferens in the man, to prevent the egg and sperm meeting. It is usually an elective procedure and should only be considered if the decision is to remain child free or if the family is considered to be complete. Full information and counselling should *always* be available to ensure that the decision is thought through, and that any worries, problems or questions can be raised and discussed. Ideally the decision to be sterilised should not be made at emotional times such as directly after childbirth, abortion or miscarriage, or when there is a relationship or personal crisis. If there are any doubts, sterilisation should not be carried out. At present both male and female sterilisation are still regarded as an irreversible procedure. Although reversals can be carried out, there is no guarantee of success. Consent from a partner for the procedure to be carried out is not required by law.

Female sterilisation

There are a number of different female sterilisation methods. The fallopian tubes which carry the egg from the ovaries to the womb can be reached either directly or indirectly:

▶ directly through an incision in the abdominal wall by laparotomy or mini-laparotomy
▶ indirectly by laparoscopy, *or* through the vagina by culdoscopy (this is not commonly used in the UK)

Laparoscopic sterilisation is the most common method today as it is simple, quick and the least invasive. Once the fallopian tubes have been reached they can be blocked by:

▶ tying and removing a small piece of tube – excision and tubal ligation
▶ sealing the tubes – cauterisation and diathermy
▶ blocking the tubes – use of clips or rings

Female sterilisation

1 Fallopian tubes cut

2 Fallopian tubes blocked

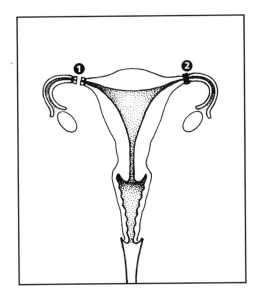

Place of operation

Female sterilisation is carried out either in hospital or in a well-equipped clinic, under a light general anaesthetic, or possibly local anaesthetic. The length of stay varies from a day to a couple of days depending on the method used.

Efficacy

Female sterilisation is highly effective, with a failure rate of 1-3 per 1000, depending on the method of sterilisation carried out. It is effective immediately.

Advantages

▶ highly effective
▶ it is effective immediately
▶ fear of unplanned pregnancy is removed
▶ it is a permanent method

Disadvantages

▶ it involves an operation and anaesthetic
▶ it is not easily reversible

Contra-indications

▶ if there are any marital or relationship problems
▶ uncertainty about the decision to be sterilised
▶ psychiatric illness
▶ a request made at a young age is a relative contra-indication (under 25)
▶ physical disability which might increase the risk of the procedure

▶ weight – gross obesity for laparoscopic procedures

▶ certain gynaecological disorders

Side-effects

There are few serious side-effects with female sterilisation and no serious long-term effects. Ovulation and menstruation continue as before. Some research suggests menstrual disturbance occurs in some women, but most research shows that sterilisation does not cause menstrual disturbance. Other factors are usually to blame, for example, age, stopping oral contraception (combined pills), or gynaecological problems such as fibroids.

Pregnancy is uncommon after sterilisation, but should it occur, there is a higher risk of ectopic pregnancy.

Psychological problems and regret are uncommon where full counselling has been available and where sterilisation is not carried out at a young age (under 25).

Sexual activity and enjoyment should not be affected, and for many it is improved as the fear of unplanned pregnancy is removed. Sexual intercourse can be resumed as soon as a woman feels comfortable. Additional contraceptive precautions are not required as female sterilisation is effective immediately.

Male sterilisation – Vasectomy

Male sterilisation (vasectomy) involves cutting or blocking the vas deferens, the tubes that carry the sperm from the testes to the penis. The vas deferens are reached via a small incision either in the middle or on each side of the scrotum. The no-scalpel technique is a refined and improved technique of vasectomy which reaches the vas deferens via a small puncture rather than an incision. A small amount of tube is removed, or cut and sealed.

Place of operation

A vasectomy is usually performed under local anaesthetic (sometimes general anaesthetic), as an outpatient

Male sterilisation

1 Vas deferens cut

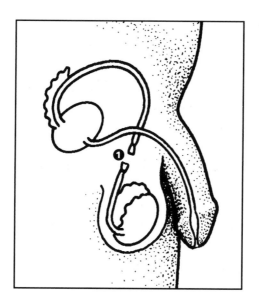

procedure in either a hospital or a well-equipped clinic or surgery. It takes about 15 minutes. It is safer and simpler than most female sterilisation.

Efficacy

Vasectomy is highly effective, with an immediate failure rate of about 1 in a 1000. Counselling should always include information about the possibility of late failure of vasectomy. It is not effective immediately: a vasectomy is considered to be effective *only* when two consecutive negative semen samples have been produced. It takes about three to four months (up to about 36 ejaculations) to clear the remaining sperm from the vas deferens. Until this occurs, an additional contraceptive method should be used at all times.

Advantages

▶ simple and easy
▶ it is safe and very effective
▶ fear of unplanned pregnancy is removed
▶ it is a permanent method

Disadvantages

▶ it is not easily reversible
▶ it is not effective immediately
▶ it involves a surgical procedure

**Contra-
indications**

▶ certain urological problems

▶ any marital or relationship problems

▶ uncertainty about the decision to be sterilised

▶ request at a young age (under 25) should be considered as a relative contraindication

▶ psychiatric illness

Side-effects

There are no effects on the male sexual organs or the male hormones. Sexual libido and functioning should not be affected. Sexual activity can be resumed as soon as a man feels comfortable. Short-term effects include possible bruising and swelling, which may last for a couple of weeks. This can be minimised by the wearing of tight underpants for a week, day and night. Heavy lifting work or vigorous sport should be avoided for at least a week.

Infection or epidymitis occurs in about 2-6 per cent of men, but this is easily treated with antibiotic therapy. Scrotal haematoma generally occurs in less than one per cent of men who have had a vasectomy. It seldom requires more than analgesia and local support.

Sperm granuloma (leakage of sperm into the tissue between the cut ends of the vas deferens) cause foreign body reaction and the formation of discrete tender nodules in about 30 per cent of vasectomies. These may cause no problems or they can cause inflammation and pain, which can easily be treated by removal.

Sperm antibodies occur in about 60-80 per cent of vasec-tomised men. (Sperm antibodies are also found less frequently in non-vasectomised men.) As sperm continue to be produced after vasectomy, they are absorbed by the body. Testicular antigens may be released into the circulation which stimulates an auto-immune response. There is no evidence that sperm antibodies impair immunity or cause any health problems.

Cardiovascular disease and vasectomy

Contrary to earlier reports suggesting a possibility of increased risk of cardiovascular disease in men after vasectomy, research has now shown this not to be the case.

Vasectomy and cancer

Worldwide about 42 million couples rely on vasectomy as their method of family planning. Studies in the 1970s and 1980s of short and long term effects of sterilisation indicated that the procedure was both effective and safe. Between 1988 and 1991, some studies suggested for the first time an increase in the risk of testicular and prostate cancer after vasectomy. The World Health Organisation (WHO) at that time concluded:

'any causal relationship between vasectomy and the risk of prostate or testicular cancer is unlikely and no change in family planning policies concerning vasectomy is justified.'

No new study has appeared to date which challenges the WHO view about testicular cancer. With regard to vasectomy and prostate cancer, two American studies published in 1993 reported an increase in the risk of prostate cancer after vasectomy. However, a third 1993 study carried out by the US National Institute of Child Health and Human Development concluded that there is no evidence that vasectomy increases the risk of auto-immune disease, arteriosclerosis or prostate cancer – at least for the first eight years or so. This carefully designed historical cohort study looked at 10,590 matched pairs.

At present family planning experts remain agreed that there is no obvious biological reason why vasectomy should be the cause of an increase in risk. The causes of prostate cancer are still not understood. This uncertainty should be raised in vasectomy counselling so clear informed decisions can be made.

As with female sterilisation, psychological problems and regret are uncommon when the decision is well thought out, and where full counselling has been available.

Reversibility of male and female sterilisation

Sterilisation is intended to be permanent. However, sometimes reversal is requested because of genuine regret or because of the death of a partner, child, or because there has been a change of relationship. A number of factors influence the success or failure of sterilisation reversal: the method used, for example clips in female sterilisation offer a better potential for reversal than methods that cut or seal the tubes; and the length of time between the operation and possible reversal. The pregnancy rate after reversal by expert surgeons can be as high as 90 per cent, but it averages between 20 and 70 per cent. Where a female sterilisation has been reversed about 3-5 per cent of pregnancies are ectopic.

Emergency contraception

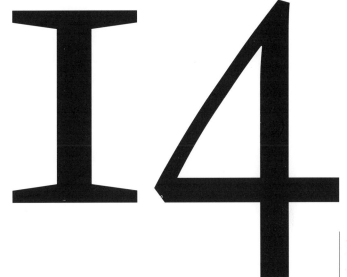

**General
information**

Emergency or postcoital contraception (originally given
the misleading name of 'morning after' contraception –
this term should now not be used) involves methods that
can be given in the event of unprotected intercourse.
Unprotected intercourse may be the result of failure to
use contraception at all, method failure, default in pill-
taking or accidents with a method. The risk of pregnancy
occurring during any day of the menstrual cycle is low.
However, at midcycle (around ovulation) the risk is about
25-30 per cent. Since it is difficult to be sure when some
women ovulate in any given cycle, the timing of giving
this treatment is not precise. Women should always
be promptly referred for treatment, even if the risk of
pregnancy is small, and in addition this provides the
opportunity to discuss future contraception. Postcoital
methods should not be used routinely.

**General mode
of action**

Postcoital methods are not abortifacients as they work
before implantation and therefore do not disrupt an
existing pregnancy. They should *not* be confused with
abortion. It is vitally important that the mode of action
is understood in order that accurate information can be
given to women considering this method. It should be
recognised that for those who believe life begins at fertilisation, as opposed to the medical and legally accepted
view that life begins at implantation, these methods may
not be acceptable.

If emergency contraception fails, research to date shows
no reported fetal abnormalities following the use of the
hormonal or IUD postcoital method. For this reason,
failed emergency contraception is not a medical indication for termination of pregnancy.

Hormonal methods

Originally, ethinyloestradiol (5mg daily for 5 days) was
used effectively for a number of years. Today lower doses
of oestrogen with a progestogen are used, as this method

has fewer side-effects when compared with the use of oestrogens alone. A combined oestrogen/progestogen formulation can be used, ie 100mcg ethinyloestradiol plus 500mcg levonorgestrel (equivalent to 2 tablets of Ovran) repeated once 12 hours later. This is known as the Yuzpe method. Schering PC4 is marketed specifically as a post-coital contraceptive.

Other hormones are being researched as postcoital methods, including progestogens and anti-progestogens such as mifepristone. Recent World Health Organisation research has suggested that the use of mifepristone may be much more effective, with fewer side-effects than the Yuzpe method, but at present mifepristone is not licensed for use as a postcoital method of contraception.

Mode of action   This is considered to be multifactorial and mainly includes:

▶ rendering the endometrium unfavourable for implantation
▶ desynchronisation of the delicate sequential effects relating to ovum transport
▶ prevention or delay in ovulation if given early enough in the cycle
▶ alteration of normal corpus luteum function which results in a shortened luteal phase

Efficacy   Effectiveness rates vary between 95 and 99 per cent.

Timing and use of hormonal methods   Hormonal methods should be given within 72 hours (3 days) of unprotected intercourse. Continued contra-ception should be advised during this time. There is no age limit, even in smokers. Treatment can be repeated in a menstrual cycle if required.

Contra-indications
▶ suspected pregnancy
▶ multiple sexual intercourse over 72 hours prior to presentation
▶ migraine at presentation in a woman with focal migraine history

▶ special care needed if past history of ectopic pregnancy

▶ breast-feeding – relative contraindication if feeding is not established

▶ past history of thrombosis – relative contraindication

Side-effects

The main side-effects are nausea and vomiting. Nausea may occur in up to 50 per cent of cases. Vomiting may occur in up to 24 per cent. An anti-emetic can be prescribed to reduce the occurrence and severity of nausea. In addition, some women experience headaches, dizziness or breast tenderness.

Women should be advised that following hormonal postcoital contraception, a period may be earlier or later than usual.

Intrauterine contraceptive devices

IUDs can be inserted as a postcoital method.

Mode of action

The presence of an IUD will prevent implantation by inducing changes in the endometrium. The copper also affects the biochemical process and enzymes involved in implantation.

Efficacy

IUDs used postcoitally are almost 100 per cent effective.

Timing of use of IUDs postcoitally

An IUD can be fitted in good faith up to five days after the earliest calculation of ovulation.

Contra-indications

▶ suspected pregnancy

▶ past history of ectopic pregnancy (relative if IUD is removed at next period)

▶ special care is needed in cases of sexual assault or unsure STD/PID histories – STD screening and/or antibiotic cover should be considered

Side-effects
- ▶ these are the same as for IUDs in general
- ▶ the possibility of a sexually transmitted infection should always be checked

General

All present methods of postcoital contraception are effective and safe. It is *essential* that full information and counselling take place *before* postcoital contraception is used, *and* good follow up arranged afterwards.

Postcoital contraception is easily available from most general practitioners or community family planning clinics.

The risks of postcoital contraception are small and are outweighed by the benefits of preventing an unwanted pregnancy.

Follow-up
All women receiving postcoital contraception should be seen at least once after using postcoital contraception. This is usually at the time of the expected period or one to two weeks later. This follow-up ensures that the method has worked and provides an opportunity to talk about future contraception.

New methods of contraception

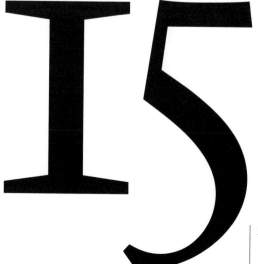

**General
information**

The idea of a new method of contraception, perhaps as big a breakthrough as the pill was in the early 1960s, always fascinates the popular press. As a result, reports that male pills, contraceptive nasal sprays, vaccines, once a month methods are 'just around the corner' have appeared repeatedly in newspapers and women's magazines, and on television during the last 25 years. As a result, health professionals may be asked about such new methods and whether they are generally available yet.

Unfortunately the answer is 'no'. Despite the hope that such methods will ultimately become available, radical new methods such as a male pill, anti-pregnancy vaccines, contraceptive nasal sprays or reversible sterilisations are at least 5, 10 or 15 years away. The time it takes for transition of a new idea to a final product can be up to 20 years or longer.

Long-acting methods are now being developed and refined. They include a range of delivery systems, including progestogen-only systems such as implants and rings, and preparations containing progestogen and oestrogen in combination, such as monthly injectables. Other methods, such as nasal sprays using gonadotrophin hormone agonists, and contraceptive vaccines are being researched.

**Contraceptive
vaginal rings**

Research is being carried out on a variety of contraceptive vaginal rings releasing progestogen or a combination of oestrogen and progestogen.

Vaginal rings are different from other long-acting hormonal methods, such as injectables and implants, because they are placed in the vagina by the woman and left there for varying lengths of time depending on the product. Being under the control of the woman, they can be removed at any time.

The most developed ring is the levonorgestrel-releasing ring; made of silicone, it lasts for 3 months. The UK vaginal ring is called Femring and will be available within the next few years.

Progestogen-releasing rings work in the same way as progestogen-only pills, with similar effectiveness rates.

Research is being carried out on several different types of ring that deliver both oestrogen and progestogen, and natural progesterone.

Pregnancy testing

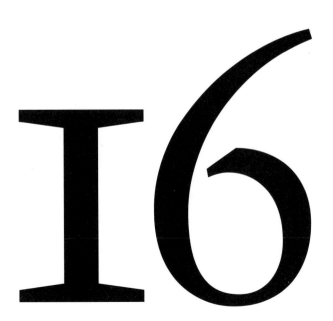

General information

Early identification of pregnancy enables improved up-take of ante-natal care and improved healthcare in early pregnancy, when the pregnancy is wanted. It facilitates the early diagnosis of fetal abnormality. In addition, and importantly, it provides time for a woman (and her partner) to make choices in the event of an unplanned pregnancy.

Pregnancy tests are carried out in a variety of places: hospitals, outpatient clinics, community family planning clinics, doctors' surgeries and pregnancy advisory centres. However, because the increase in control of expenditure in NHS hospitals and changes in services offered by doctors, pregnancy testing is becoming more difficult to obtain quickly and easily on the NHS. So many pharmacies now offer a pregnancy testing service and sell 'home pregnancy testing kits'.

Pregnancy testing *should* be readily available on request in general practitioners' surgeries and in community family planning clinics. Some GPs and clinics send pregnancy tests to local laboratories, which may mean waiting longer for the result. Many practices now undertake pregnancy testing on the premises. Good counselling should always be available with a pregnancy testing service.

Pregnancy testing in pharmacies

Pregnancy testing is a professional service offered by many community pharmacists. The following guidelines have been issued by the Council of the Royal Pharmaceutical Society who operate a strict code of practice:

Confidentiality

The pharmacist must keep all information provided by the patient and the result of the test confidential and only disclose information with the consent of the patient.

Facilities for carrying out the test

A reliable method of testing should be used. It is important that care is taken to prevent contamination which can be caused by the handling of samples of urine. This should be achieved by the use of a room separate from that used for dispensing. This should be maintained in a clean and tidy condition and all working surfaces should be finished with a smooth, impervious and washable material. Adequate lighting should be provided so that the results of the test can be read correctly. A separate sink should be provided.

Procedures which ensure that no confusion occurs between samples must be devised and followed.

Persons carrying out tests should wash their hands before leaving the working area.

All cuts and grazes on hands or on exposed parts of the body must be covered with waterproof dressings.

Request for a pregnancy test

A signed and dated confirmation of the request should be obtained. The form on which confirmation is obtained should state the limits of accuracy of the test. All questions relating to the test should be asked by the pharmacist and the answers recorded in writing.

Records

A written record of the result of the test, together with information provided by the patient and the type of test and batch number of the test materials, should be retained by the pharmacist for at least one year. Such records must be stored safely to preserve confidentiality.

Communication of the result

The result of the test should be provided in writing on a standard form. If it is necessary to convey the result by telephone, the pharmacist should be satisfied that the person requesting the information is the person who requested the test.

A written confirmation of the result should be provided even when the result has been communicated by telephone.

The form should be dated and give the name and address of the patient. The result should be given as positive *or negative with an explanation of such terms and the limits of accuracy of the test. At the request of the patient, a copy of the form should be sent to her medical practitioner. Notwithstanding the result of the test, the patient should be strongly advised to consult her medical practitioner or, if she appears reluctant to do so, another source of medical advice, eg a pregnancy advisory bureau. The pharmacist should not recommend a particular pregnancy advisory bureau but should have a list available for use if the patient requests information.*

Advice from the pharmacist

The pharmacist can clearly provide invaluable support in this area, especially if a woman is undecided or ambivalent about the pregnancy, as many are. The pharmacist can provide appropriate information to refer the woman immediately for counselling and medical help. Many pharmacists have set aside quieter, more discreet areas where discussion can be relatively private.

Home pregnancy tests

The vast majority of pharmacists sell 'do-it-yourself pregnancy testing kits' such as Discover, First Response and Clear Blue One Step, or their own brands. These pregnancy tests are about 99 per cent accurate if the instructions are carried out correctly. Today, such pregnancy tests can be used from the first day of a missed period.

False results

False negative results

Home pregnancy tests may be difficult to carry out, especially if a woman is nervous about the outcome of the test. False negative results are much more likely than false positives with all kinds of pregnancy tests. False negative results can be due to:

▶ too little, too dilute, or too old urine
▶ traces of detergent in the urine container
▶ reading the test too soon
▶ disturbing the test

A false negative result can also be due to medical causes, such as ectopic pregnancy or a threatened miscarriage.

False positive results

False positive results can be due to:

▶ raised hCG for reasons other than pregnancy
▶ raised gonadotrophins around the menopause
▶ badly performed tests
▶ heavy proteinuria or haematuria
▶ contamination with soap or detergent
▶ certain drugs

Problems in early pregnancy

Now that pregnancy can be confirmed so early, there is a greater awareness of miscarriage, and the fact that many pregnancies do not go to term. About 15-20 per cent of pregnancies are lost in the first 3 months, often at the time when a period would have been due, ie at 2 or 3 months from the date of the last menstrual period. Any woman who has any bleeding and/or lower abdominal pain early in pregnancy should be referred without delay. Such a pregnancy may continue, be miscarried or be ectopic. Ectopic pregnancy occurs in 1.2-1.4 per cent of all pregnancies, and accounts for up to 10 per cent of maternal mortality.

Abortion

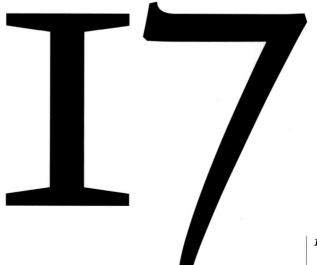

Abortion is not considered to be a method of contraception, however it is an important and necessary back-up to family planning services.

The Abortion Act 1967

Before 1967 abortion was legal only to save the life of the mother. The 1967 Abortion Act extended the grounds for legal abortion in England, Wales and Scotland. It does not apply to Northern Ireland.

Under the act, legal termination of pregnancy may be carried out provided that two registered medical practitioners agree that it is necessary on one or more of the following grounds:

▶ the continuance of the pregnancy would involve risk to the life of the pregnant woman, or of injury to her physical or mental health, or that of any existing children, greater than if the pregnancy were terminated
▶ there is substantial risk of the child being born handicapped

In determining the risk of injury to health of the woman or her children, the woman's actual or reasonably foreseeable future environment may be taken into account. No person is obliged to perform or participate in an abortion to which they have a conscientious objection. If the pregnant woman is married, her husband's consent, though desirable, is not obligatory. If she is under 16 her parents should be consulted except in exceptional circumstances when it is left to the doctor's clinical judgment.

In an emergency, one doctor may decide to perform the operation to save the life of the woman or to protect her from grave permanent injury.

Abortion services are controlled by Department of Health regulations. Except in an emergency, abortion may take place only in an NHS hospital or in a private nursing home approved for this purpose by the Department of Health.

This includes the administration of the abortifacient, mifepristone.

1990 Amendment to the 1967 Abortion Act

The Abortion Act 1967 is now amended by Section 37 of the Human Fertilisation and Embryology Act. The amendment does not modify the general principles of the original act, and does not alter the basis of access to abortion. The amendment covers three areas:

▶ It introduces a new upper time limit of 24 weeks for legal abortion, although no upper time limit applies in a few very extreme specified circumstances. These are:
▷ risk to the life of the mother
▷ risk of grave permanent injury to the mother
▷ risk of serious fetal handicap

▶ It brings selective induced miscarriage in a multiple pregnancy under the terms of the Abortion Act 1967.

▶ It authorises the Secretary of State for Health to approve a new class of places for the purposes of medical termination of pregnancy. This prepares the way for the licensing of places appropriate to methods of abortion using drugs.

Public opinion and views

Successive opinion polls make it clear that the majority of British people support the 1967 Act. A Harris poll conducted in 1991 for the Abortion Law Reform Association found that 81 per cent of those questioned thought that women should have the right to chose an abortion in the first three months of pregnancy. The annual British Social Attitudes Survey reveals that in the 1980s attitudes became significantly more liberal towards the social and medical grounds for abortion. These views have not changed in the 1990s.

Availability

There is no legal requirement for health authorities to provide an abortion service. The level of provision varies considerably between districts from very good to extremely poor.

Charitable abortion clinics within the private sector developed after the 1967 Act was passed, to meet needs which could not be met by the NHS at that time. The continuing importance of private sector abortions largely reflects continuing inadequacies in NHS provision for abortion.

Private abortion clinics have to be classed as approved places for termination of pregnancy and are closely regulated by the Department of Health.

Counselling

Pregnancy counselling should always be available for women who have an unplanned pregnancy. Informed, non-directive counselling allows a woman (and her partner) to be sure of any decision made with regard to continuing or terminating a pregnancy.

Methods of abortion

Surgical techniques

In practice, most abortions are carried out within the first 12 weeks of pregnancy (first trimester). Up to this time abortions can be carried out safely by simple techniques such as vacuum aspiration or dilatation and curettage (D&C).

▶ Vacuum aspiration

In vacuum aspiration, the cervix is dilated and the womb is emptied by suction through a thin plastic tube, and the procedure is usually carried out under light general anaesthetic or less usually under local anaesthetic.

▶ Dilatation and curettage (D&C)

D&C involves dilating the cervix and introducing a curette into the womb to remove the contents. It is carried out under general anaesthetic.

Abortions carried out after 12 weeks (second trimester abortions) can be more difficult, with a higher complication rate. There are two methods:

▶ Dilatation and evacuation (D&E)

In a D&E, the cervix is dilated and the contents of the womb – fetus and placenta – are removed with special forceps. The uterus is further emptied by vacuum aspiration. It is carried out under general anaesthetic. This method can be used up to 20 weeks, but most hospitals prefer to use medical induction after 16 weeks.

▶ Medical induction

Medical induction involves inducing labour: usually prostaglandin is administered by vaginal pessary or injections. Drugs used to stimulate labour at full term can also be used. The fetus is expelled. Late abortions are carried out infrequently.

Medical methods

Anti-progestogens

Anti-progestogens work by blocking the action of progesterone which is necessary for the maintenance of the pregnancy.

The use of mifepristone marketed by Roussel as Mifegyne, provides a medical alternative for some women to the presently available surgical techniques of abortion. This method can be used in the first 9 weeks of pregnancy (63 days from the first day of the last period) and involves the use of mifepristone, with a prostaglandin. It is highly effective.

Legal and ethical issues

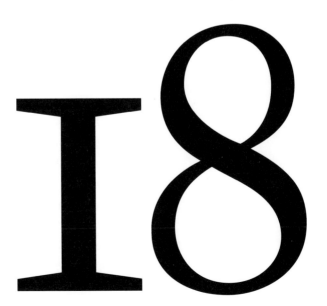

**General
information**

The Family Law Reform Act 1969 (Section 8) in England
provides that the consent to medical or surgical treatment
of an individual who has attained the age of 16 shall be
effective consent, and that in such cases it is not necessary
to obtain consent from a parent or guardian. The medical
age of consent in Scotland is 16, and it is 17 in Northern
Ireland. In general, family planning services, methods and
supplies are available to all, irrespective of age, sex or
marital status. However, there are special guidelines for
young people.

For a full review see FPA Factsheet 5F *Some laws on sex*.

Under-16s

The provision of written or verbal information, services
or prescription of family planning methods to under-16s
is legal without parental consent in England, Scotland
and Wales (and to under-17s in Northern Ireland).

Public attention in England was drawn to the dilemmas
concerning contraception and the under-16s by the
'Gillick' case.

The decision whether or not to prescribe contraception
for a person under 16 without parental consent ultimately
rests with the clinical judgment of the doctor.

Specific advice and guidance is provided to doctors, health
authorities and other health professionals by the Department of Health in their 1986 circular *Family planning
services for young people*. (This updates Section G of the
Family planning service memorandum of guidance 1974).
This circular relates only to England and Wales. The
equivalent Scottish circular, the *National health circular
(gen) 5* makes no mention of the under-16s, but provides
advice that services should be available to all. In Northern
Ireland the situation regarding the under-17s is the same
as that applying in England to the under-16s. The Department of Health's guidance to doctors and health professionals includes the following advice:

▶ In considering the provision of advice or treatment on contraception doctors and other professional staff need to take special care not to undermine parental responsibility and family stability. The doctor or other professional should therefore always seek to persuade the young person to tell the parents or guardian (or other person in loco parentis), or to let him or her inform them that advice or treatment is given. It should be most unusual for a doctor or other professional to provide advice or treatment in relation to contraception to a young person under 16 without parental knowledge or consent.

▶ Exceptionally, there will be cases where it is not possible to persuade the young person either to inform the parents or to allow the doctor or other professional to do so. This may be, for example, where family relationships have broken down. In such cases, a doctor or other professional would be justified in giving advice and treatment without parental knowledge or consent, provided they were satisfied:

▷ that the young person could understand the advice and had sufficient maturity to understand what was involved in terms of the moral, social and emotional implications
▷ that they could neither persuade the young person to inform the parents, nor to allow him/her to inform them, that contraceptive advice was being sought
▷ that the young person would be very likely to begin, or to continue having, sexual intercourse with or without contraceptive treatment
▷ that, without contraceptive advice or treatment, the young person's physical or mental health, or both, would be likely to suffer
▷ that the young person's best interests required them to give contraceptive advice, treatment or both without parental consent

For a full review, refer to FPA Factsheet 5E, *The legal position regarding contraceptive advice and provision to young people.*

New guidance clarifying the position about confidentiality and under-16s has been issued jointly by the BMA, GMSC, Brook, FPA and the RCGP (see 'Recommended reading' on page 160).

Reproductive health care services

19

General information

All addresses of organisations listed in this chapter can be found under 'Addresses of useful organisations' on pages 151-159.

Contraception is an important part of family planning, but as discussed there are many other health issues within the area of family planning. People may well raise related issues such as planning for a family or having a healthy pregnancy, concern about sexually transmitted diseases, the menopause etc. It is helpful if professionals can provide information and addresses of services and refer the person to an appropriate source of help.

Youth advisory services

Some NHS clinics have special sessions for young people. Details of these clinics may be obtained from the FPA. Brook Advisory Centres welcome under-25s. In major cities there may be special youth advisory centres providing family planning services, counselling, help and support about all personal and relationship problems.

Brook Advisory Centres

These are family planning clinics providing special services for young people (mainly under-25s) which were set up in 1964. They help with any contraception advice and supplies, help with any sexual, emotional or relationship problem and provide pregnancy testing and pregnancy counselling. Most services are free, but a fee is payable at some clinics. There are clinics in Birmingham, Bristol, Edinburgh, London, Merseyside, Burnley, Milton Keynes, Birkenhead, Telford, Salford, Cornwall and Northern Ireland. Brook also produces educational aids and literature. Central office address:
153A East Street
London SE17 2SD
☎ 071 708 1234

Sexually transmitted diseases including HIV

Any person concerned or worried about a possible sexually transmitted infection, including HIV, should receive help and advice or be referred to a genito-urinary medicine clinic (GUM clinic). In the UK, the Venereal Disease Regulations (1916) allowed for the establishment of clinics for the diagnosis and treatment *in confidence* of sexually transmitted diseases. In addition to diagnosis and treatment, trained counsellors and health advisers are available to provide information, help and support. GUM clinics can be found attached to most large hospitals.

Contraception and STDs

Contraceptive methods, in addition to preventing unplanned pregnancy, can in some cases protect against STDs. Until recently, contraceptive technology development, policy emphasis and service delivery have focused mainly on preventing pregnancy, with little attention being paid to prevention of STDs. In the UK, services for providing contraception are entirely separate from those services for diagnosis and treatment of STDs – they are financed from different budgets, situated in separate buildings and run by staff with a different approach, training and career structure. However, more recently the need for collaboration has been recognised with some GUM clinics now having a family planning session or employing staff with additional family planning training. Studies show that many women attending GUM clinics require contraceptive advice and those attending family planning clinics need advice on STDs. Some areas of the country are now developing sexual health services instead of separate family planning and STD services.

There are a number of organisations and groups set up to help people concerned or worried about HIV and AIDS (see 'Addresses of useful organisations' on page 158).

The FPA can provide details of UK GUM clinic services.

Sexual problems

Individuals or couples with sexual difficulties can seek professional help about psychosexual counselling. Some NHS community family planning clinics hold psychosexual sessions, which may need a GP referral. Some GPs are also trained to provide the service.

The FPA can help with enquiries about services within the UK. The Institute of Psychosexual Medicine can also help with enquiries about practitioners trained in psycho-sexual medicine.

Relationship/ marriage problems

Counselling and help may be obtained from:

► RELATE
► Catholic Marriage Advisory Council
► Jewish Marriage Education Council

Well-woman services

Well-woman services exists to provide screening for breast and cervical cancer, instruction in breast self-examination, blood pressure checks etc, in symptom-free women.

Well-man services

Well-man services exist in a few areas and provide general health screening.

Cervical smears and breast checks

Cervical smears are performed by general practitioners, or practice nurses in GP surgeries or as part of a contra-ceptive service at family planning clinics. A woman should have a cervical smear every three to five years once sexually active. Breast checks are also carried out routinely at family planning clinics and as necessary by family doctors. Women over 50 are recommended to have routine breast screening (mammography) every three years. Women should be encouraged to be aware of their breasts and therefore aware of any changes. Leaflets are available from the Women's Nationwide Cancer Control Campaign (WNCCC), The Breast Care and Mastectomy Association (BCMA) and BACUP.

Those seeking well-women services without contracep-tive advice can go to a well-woman clinic without referral by a GP. These clinics are run by many district health authorities as part of the community services. Some private clinics also exist. Addresses of well-woman clinics can be obtained from the FPA.

Pre-pregnancy care

Pre-pregnancy care can help women and their partners to prepare for pregnancy both physically and psychologically. It also provides an opportunity for health professionals to give advice in this area. Issues such as nutrition, diet, rubella, exercise, smoking, health and work should be addressed.

Infertility

About 10-15 per cent of couples are infertile, this being defined as pregnancy not occurring after one year of trying for a baby. Considerable unhappiness may be experienced by a couple who find themselves infertile. There is often a feeling of isolation among those who have a fertility problem, as they may feel that no one else can understand their problem.

Two main organisations are available to help with this problem in the UK:

▶ ISSUE
▶ CHILD

There are also a number of hospital fertility units which provide support groups.

Premenstrual syndrome

The premenstrual syndrome (PMS) is characterised by a group of symptoms which may occur in the second half of a woman's menstrual cycle just before her period. These symptoms which vary from woman to woman include depression, irritability, headaches, fluid retention and tiredness. Today there is a better understanding of PMS and this has led to improved forms of help and treatment.

Women should be encouraged to seek help from their GP. Some family planning clinics provide help. There are a few NHS specialist PMS clinics. The organisation PREMSOC can help with advice and support.

Menopause

The menopause or change of life is the time when a woman's periods finally cease. Cyclical changes in hormone output may be disturbed for several months before the menopause, and women may experience symptoms due to oestrogen deficiency for some time after their periods cease. Not all women find the menopause a troublesome time in life; many pass smoothly through it. Others are disabled by certain symptoms and require help and advice.

Menopausal symptoms include hot flushes or cold sweats, numbness and tingling, vaginal dryness, nervousness and irritability, depression and poor sleep.

Women seeking help should be referred to their own doctor in the first instance or to a menopause clinic. Women's Health Concern can provide help and advice. The Menopause Society can provide advice for professionals.

The FPA can provide information on menopause clinics in the UK.

Contraception and the menopause

The recommended medical guidelines from the Medical Advisory Committees of the FPA and the Faculty of Family Planning and Reproductive Health Care are that contra-ceptive methods should be continued until a woman has not had a period or any bleeding for two years if she is aged under 50, or one year if she is over 50.

Note

See 'Addresses of useful organisations ' on page 159.

Family planning training

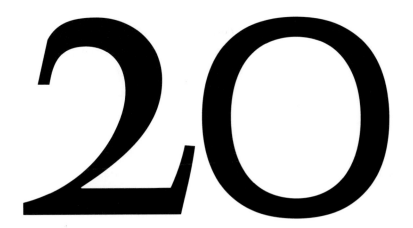

Clinical training

Fertility and reproductive health issues are now a recognised part of undergraduate medical training. However, specific family planning training is minimal. Doctors and nurses providing family planning should hold a recognised family planning qualification such as the UK Joint Committee on Contraception (JCC) certificate in family planning for doctors (from 1993, the Faculty of Family Planning and Reproductive Health Care Diploma) or the recognised family planning certificates from the English, Scottish, Northern Ireland or Welsh National Boards of Nursing.

Training in psychosexual medicine

The Institute of Psychosexual Medicine provides training and research in this area. It offers training to doctors to improve their skills with clients who seek help with sexual difficulties. A certificate of competence is issued after completion of recognised courses of instruction.

The Association of Sexual and Marital Therapists provides research, training and skills to medical and health professionals.

Non-clinical training

Family planning is not primarily a medical issue. The role of a family planning service is to empower clients to take responsibility for, and exercise choice over, their sexual and reproductive health, and to provide support for those experiencing difficulties in relation to their sexuality. While the provision of contraception clearly requires medical knowledge and skills, a comprehensive family planning service is as much about non-medical health education and health promotion and the provision of advice, information and counselling.

Training about sexuality in all its aspects and in counselling, communication and active listening skills is essential. The FPA has worked with key family planning providers for over 60 years and has extensive experience in providing training about sexuality and communication to professionals, and in responding to the information needs of the general public as well as providers of family planning and sexual health services. This experience confirms the need for all working in the field of sexual health and family planning to undertake, in addition to appropriate clinical training, experiential training that involves sexuality, exploration of values and attitudes and development of communication skills.

The FPA is committed to supporting the development of family planning services and provides communication and sexuality training for health and medical professionals.

Addresses of useful organisations

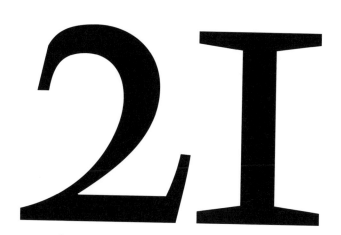

**The FPA in
the UK**

The Family Planning Association
27-35 Mortimer Street
London WIN 7RJ
☎ 071 636 7866

The FPA in Wales
4 Museum Place
Cardiff CFI 3BG
☎ 0222 342766

The FPA in Northern Ireland
113 University Street
Belfast BT7 IHP
☎ 0232 325488

The FPA in Scotland
Scottish centre to be re-opened in 1994

**The health
promotion
agencies of
the UK**

The Health Education Authority
Hamilton House
Mabledon Place
London WCIH 9TX
☎ 071 383 3833

The Health Education Board for Scotland
Woodburn House
Canaan Lane
Edinburgh EHIO 4SF
☎ 031 447 8044

Health Promotion Wales
Ffynnon-las
Ty Glas Avenue
Llanishen
Cardiff CF4 5DZ
☎ 0222 752222

The Health Promotion Agency for Northern Ireland
23 Hampton Park
Belfast BT7 3JW
☎ 0232 644811

Medical and family planning organisations

British Medical Association
BMA House
Tavistock Square
London WC1H 9JP
☎ 071 387 4499

Faculty of Family Planning and Reproductive Health Care of the RCOG
27 Sussex Place
Regent's Park
London NW1 4RG
☎ 071 262 5425

National Association of Family Planning Doctors
now the Faculty of Family Planning and Reproductive Health Care (see above)

National Association of Family Planning Nurses
c/o EMY Secretarial Services
19 Whiteacre Road
Knowle
Solihull
West Midlands B93 9HW
☎ 0564 770032

RCN FP Forum
Royal College of Nursing
20 Cavendish Square
London W1M 9AE
☎ 071 409 3333

Royal College of General Practitioners
14 Princes Gate
London SW7 1PU
☎ 071 581 3232

The Margaret Pyke Centre
15 Batemans Buildings
Soho Square
London WIV 5TW
☎ 071 734 9351

The Royal Pharmaceutical Society of Great Britain
1 Lambeth High Street
London SE1 7JN
☎ 071 735 9141

Natural family planning organisations

The Natural Family Planning Service of the Catholic Marriage Advisory Council
Clitherow House
1 Blythe Mews
Blythe Road
London W14 0NW
☎ 071 371 1341

National Association of Natural Family Planning Teachers (NANFPT)
Natural Family Planning Centre
Birmingham Maternity Hospital
Edgbaston
Birmingham B15 2TG
☎ 021 472 3806

Training (in family planning for doctors and nurses)

Faculty of Family Planning and Reproductive Health Care
27 Sussex Place
Regent's Park
London NW1 4RG
☎ 071 262 5425

English National Board for Nursing
Victory House
170 Tottenham Court Road
London W1P 0HA
☎ 071 388 3131

Welsh National Board for Nursing
Floor 13
Pearl Assurance House
Grey Friars Road
Cardiff CF1 3AG
☎ 0222 395535

National Board for Nursing for Scotland
22 Queen Street
Edinburgh EH2 1JX
☎ 031 226 7371

National Board for Nursing for Northern Ireland
RAC House
79 Chichester Street
Belfast BT1 4JE
☎ 0232 238152

Young people

Brook Advisory Centres
(Head Office)
153A East Street
London SE17 2SD
☎ 071 708 1234

Abortion

Birth Control Trust
27-35 Mortimer Street
London W1N 7RJ
☎ 071 580 9360

Pregnancy charities

British Pregnancy Advisory Service (BPAS)
Austy Manor
Wootton Warren
Solihull
West Midlands B95 6BX
☎ 0564 793225

Marie Stopes House
108 Whitfield Street
London W1P 6BE
☎ 071 388 0662

Relationships

RELATE
Herbert Gray College
Little Church Street
Rugby
Warwickshire CV21 3AP
☎ 0788 573241

Jewish Marriage Education Council
23 Ravenshurst Avenue
London NW4 4EL
☎ 071 203 6311

Catholic Marriage Advisory Council
Clitherow House
1 Blythe Mews
Blythe Road
London W14 0NW
☎ 071 371 1341

Infertility

ISSUE (The National Fertility Association)
509 Aldridge Road
Great Barr
Birmingham B44 8NA
☎ 021 344 4414

CHILD
Suite 219
Caledonian House
98 The Centre
Feltham
Middlesex TW13 4BH
☎ 081 893 7110

Sexual identity issues

The Albany Trust
The Sunra Centre
26 Balham Hill
London SW12 9EB
☎ 081 675 6669

Lesbian and gay support

Gay Switchboard
BM Switchboard
London WC1N 3XX
☎ 071 837 7324

Women's Health
52 Featherstone Street
London EC1Y 8RT
☎ 071 251 6580

One parent families

National Council for One Parent Families
255 Kentish Town Road
London NW5 2LX
☎ 071 267 1361

Cancer organisations

BACUP (British Association of Cancer United Patients)
3 Bath Place
Rivington Street
London EC2A 3JR
☎ 071 613 2121

Women's Nationwide Cancer Control Campaign (WNCCC)
Suna House
128-30 Curtain Road
London EC2 3AR
☎ 071 729 2229

Breast Care & Mastectomy Association
15-19 Britten Street
London SW3 3TZ
☎ 071 867 1103

STDs including HIV/AIDS

For details about NHS genito-urinary medicine (GUM) services, contact the FPA information helpline, on ☎ 071 636 7866 (Monday to Friday, 10am to 3pm)

National AIDS Trust
6th Floor
Eileen House
80 Newington Causeway
London SE1 6AF
☎ 071 972 2845

National AIDS Helpline
☎ 0800 567123

Terence Higgins Trust
BM AIDS
London WC1N 3XX
☎ 071 242 1010 (helpline)
☎ 071 831 0330 (administration)

Pregnancy organisations

Maternity Alliance
15 Britannia Street
London WC1X 9JP
☎ 071 837 1265

National Childbirth Trust
Alexandra House
Oldham Terrace
London W3 6NH
☎ 081 992 8637

Miscarriage Association
Clayton Hospital
Northgate
Wakefield
West Yorkshire WF1 8JS
☎ 0924 200799

PMS support	**PREMSOC** PO Box 102 London SE1 7ES
Menopause support	**Women's Health Concern** PO Box 1629 London W8 6AU ☎ 071 938 3932
	The British Menopause Society 36 West Street Marlow Buckinghamshire SO7 2NB ☎ 0628 890199
Psychosexual problems	**Institute of Psychosexual Medicine** 11 Chandos Street London W1M 9DE ☎ 071 580 0631
	Association of Sexual and Marital Therapists Box 62 Sheffield 10
General women's health	**Women's Health** 52 Featherstone Street London EC1Y 8RT ☎ 071 251 6580

Recommended reading

Contraception and family planning

▶ *Contraception and sexuality in health and disease*
Sapire, K Esther
(UK edition revised and updated by T Belfield and
J Guillebaud)
McGraw Hill 1990

▶ *Handbook of family planning*
Loudon, N (ed)
2nd edn, Churchill Livingstone 1991

▶ *Contraception – your questions answered*
Guillebaud, J
2nd edn, Churchill Livingstone 1993

▶ *RCN guidelines for domiciliary family planning*
RCN 1993

▶ *Confidentiality and people under 16*
A guidance note issued jointly by the BMA, GMSC,
Brook Advisory Centres, FPA and RCGP
BMA 1993

▶ *Pharmacokinetic drug interactions with oral
contraceptives*
Back, D J and Orme, M L E
Clinical Pharmacokinetics, vol 18, no 6, pp 472-81, 1990

▶ *Fertility: a comprehensive guide to natural family
planning*
Chubb, E and Knight, J
2nd edn, David and Charles 1992

▶ *Directory of hormonal contraceptives*
Kleinman, R
2nd edn, IPPF 1992

▶ *Emergency (postcoital) contraception: guidelines for doctors*
National Association of Family Planning Doctors
British Journal of Family Planning, vol 18, no 3, 1992
(see also Erratum, BJFP vol 18, no 4, 1992)

▶ *Long-term use of copper intrauterine devices*
A statement from the Medical Advisory Committee of the FPA and NAFPD
The Lancet, 2 June 1990, pp 1322-3

▶ **Sexuality and birth control in community work**
Christopher, E
2nd edn, Tavistock 1987

Sexually transmitted diseases

▶ **ABC of sexually transmitted diseases**
Adler, H
2nd edn, BMA 1990

▶ **Sexually transmitted diseases**
Csonka, GW et al
Balliere Tindall 1990

Sexuality

▶ **Introduction to psychosexual medicine**
Skrine, R L
Chapman and Hall 1989

▶ **Human sexuality and its problems**
Bancroft, J
2nd edn, Churchill Livingstone 1989

▶ **Contraceptive care – meeting individual needs**
Montford, H and Skrine, R (eds)
Chapman and Hall 1993

Hormonal replacement therapy

▶ **Hormone replacement therapy – your questions answered**
Whitehead, M and Godfree, V
Churchill Livingstone 1992

General

▶ *Handbook of pharmacy health education*
Martin, J (ed)
The Pharmaceutical Press 1991

▶ *Women's problems in general practice*
McPherson, A (ed)
3rd edn, Oxford University Press 1993

FPA publications and FPA helpline

The FPA has developed a unique range of publications for professionals and consumers in the areas of sexuality, sex education and contraception.

Publications for consumers

▶ *FPA consumer leaflets on contraceptive methods*

▶ *FPA sexual health booklets*

▶ *The FPA guide to contraception*
Hayman, S
Thorsons 1993

Publications for professionals

The FPA produces training resources, teaching materials, reference guides, factsheets and a regular news bulletin - for health professionals in a range of settings.

▶ *Contraceptive display kit*
(Sample contraceptives, leaflets and teacher's manual)
FPA 1992

▶ *Contraceptive handbook: a reference guide to family planning methods and services for pharmacists*
Belfield, T
3rd edn, FPA 1992

▶ *Family Planning Today*
A quarterly bulletin for family planning and health professionals

▶ *FPA factfile*
A series of 21 factsheets on contraception, sexuality and sex education

Details of these and over 800 other publications on sexuality and contraception are available from Healthwise, the FPA's bookshop and mail order service. For a catalogue, please send a stamped addressed envelope to **Healthwise**

27-35 Mortimer Street

London WIN 7RJ

FPA helpline

The FPA runs a nationwide information line for professionals and members of the general public who have enquiries on contraception, fertility and other issues relating to sexual health. It can also provide details of all UK family planning clinics and other reproductive health services. Call on any weekday from 10am to 3pm, or write, with SAE, to the Information Department at the address above.

FPA helpline ☎ 071 636 7866

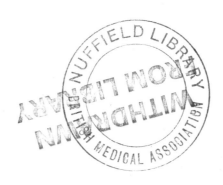